Practical Prescribing Guidelines in Rheumatoid Arthritis

Practical Prescribing Guidelines in Rheumatoid Arthritis

Edited by

Hilary Capell, MD, FRCP

Rajan Madhok, MD, FRCP

Iain B. McInnes, PhD, MRCP

Centre for Rheumatic Diseases
Glasgow Royal Infirmary
Scotland, UK

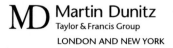
Martin Dunitz
Taylor & Francis Group
LONDON AND NEW YORK

© 2003 Martin Dunitz, an imprint of the Taylor & Francis Group

First published in the United Kingdom in 2003
by Martin Dunitz, an imprint of the Taylor & Francis Group, 11 New Fetter Lane,
London EC4P 4EE

Tel.:   +44 (0) 20 7583 9855
Fax.:   +44 (0) 20 7842 2298
E-mail: info@dunitz.co.uk
Website: http://www.dunitz.co.uk

A CIP record for this book is available from the British Library.

ISBN 1–84184–282–6

Distributed in the USA by
Fulfilment Center
Taylor & Francis
10650 Tobben Drive
Independence, KY 41051, USA
Toll Free Tel.:   +1 800 634 7064
E-mail: taylorandfrancis@thomsonlearning.com

Distributed in Canada by
Taylor & Francis
74 Rolark Drive
Scarborough, Ontario M1R 4G2, Canada
Toll Free Tel.:   +1 877 226 2237
E-mail: tal_fran@istar.ca

Distributed in the rest of the world by
Thomson Publishing Services
Cheriton House
North Way
Andover, Hampshire SP10 5BE, UK

Tel.:   +44 (0)1264 332424
E-mail: salesorder.tandf@thomsonpublishingservices.co.uk

Composition by Wearset Ltd, Boldon, Tyne and Wear

Printed and bound in Great Britain by The Cromwell Press, Trowbridge.

Contents

Contributors

The editors are grateful to a number of colleagues for their contributions to this text.

Peter Brooks wrote the introductory section on NSAIDs.

Maciej Brzeski wrote the section on cyclophosphamide.

WW Buchanan wrote the introductory section on history, epidemiology and assessment of response.

Max Field wrote the section on hydroxychloroquine.

John Hunter co-wrote the sections on azathioprine and chlorambucil.

Sarah Irvine co-wrote the section on sodium aurothiomalate.

David Kane wrote the section on cyclosporin.

John Larkin co-wrote the introductory section on NSAIDs.

Dorothy Mason was the Pharmacy Advisor.

David McCarey wrote the section on minocycline.

Anne McEntegart wrote the section on leflunomide.

Lisa McKenzie co-wrote the sections on azathioprine and chlorambucil.

Elaine Morrison wrote the chapter on corticosteroids.

Robin Munro wrote the section on penicillamine.

Duncan Porter wrote the section on methotrexate.

Tom Pullar wrote the section on auranofin.

Roger Sturrock co-wrote the section on sodium aurothiomalate.

1 INTRODUCTION

Is there no balm in Gilead?
Is there no physician there?
Jeremiah VIII, 22

The balm of Gilead and the electuaries, mithridatium and therica, testify to the antiquity of therapeutics. The Biblical balm of Gilead was a resin extracted from the balsam tree and used as a counter-irritant to relieve pain (Rosner 1993). Mithridatium is ascribed to King Mithridates VI of Pontus in Asia Minor in the first century BC, and therica was the invention of Andromachus, physician to the Emperor Nero a century later (Watson 1993). Both these remedies became so popular that they were regarded as virtual panaceas. It was William Heberden, the Elder (1710–1801) of digital joint node fame, who was the first to denounce the "farago" of nonsense in a reasoned attack published as a short essay in 1745 (Heberden 1929). However, it was not until 1788 that these concoctions were removed from the London Pharmacopoeia, and not until 1884 from the last of the European Pharmacopoeias, that of France. Heberden, however, introduced his own form of therica, known as *Mistura Ferri Aromatica* and popularly as Heberden's ink, which remained in the British Pharmacopoeia until 1890 (Buchanan and Kean 1987).

It might be thought that such therapies were of the forgotten past, but the reverse is the case. During the past decades there has been a continuing rise in complementary medicine. In a 1997 survey in the United States 42% of 2055 adult responders reported using some type of alternative therapy during the previous year (Eisenberg *et al.* 1998). Such therapy has been shown to contain various contaminants, which may be harmful (Goldman and Myerson 1991; Shaw 1998; Ernst 1998).

There is an urgent need to codify information regarding herbal medicines, and if not to evaluate their benefits clinically at least to indicate their side-effects and potential interactions with conventional drugs. Patients who are receiving the disease-modifying antirheumatic drug methotrexate require to be warned that herbal supplements or other preparations they might take could, like ethanol, lead to liver damage.

Most orthodox physicians consider complementary medicines as merely placebos (Joyce 1994). However, some have been shown to be therapeutically effective, one classic example being oral extract of white willow bark (*Salix alba*). This has recently been shown in a randomized double-blind trial to be effective in treating exacerbations of low back pain (Chrubasik *et al.* 2000). This would be ascribed to salicin, which is biotransformed to salicylic acid (Schmid *et al.* 2001), but the daily doses of the administered willow bark were of the order of 120 mg and 240 mg salicin, which is equivalent to only 25 mg and 50 mg of acetylsalicylic acid. This amount of salicin cannot explain the results, and there is evidence that other analgesic and anti-inflammatory agents may be responsible (Rice-Evans *et al.* 1995; Rohnert *et al.* 1998; Guyatt *et al.* 1990).

■ ASSESSMENT OF EFFICACY AND TOXICITY OF ANTIRHEUMATIC DRUGS

With the ever-increasing number of new antirheumatic drugs, and the appreciation that clinical impressions can be misleading, the randomized placebo-controlled clinical therapeutic trial has gained acceptance as the most powerful design for assessing effectiveness of therapy. The quality of many therapeutic trials of antirheumatic drugs leaves little ground for complacency, hence an outline of design and statistical interpretation seems appropriate.

There are nine basic components to a clinical trial, namely: research objective; trial design; sample size calculation; patient selection; randomization and stratification; intervention, co-intervention, contamination and compliance; outcome assessment; statistical analysis; and interpretation.

Research objective
Although there is a great temptation to seek answers to multiple questions and to dredge data *a posteriori*, the best trials are those that are designed to answer one or at the most two questions.

Trial design
There are five types of trial design: randomized parallel; randomized crossover; sequential; nonrandomized comparative group; and one-group noncomparative open design. Parallel groups generally require larger numbers of patients than crossover studies, but the latter often present difficulties with carry-over effects, especially with drugs with a long plasma half-life. The n-of-1 trial is a variation of the crossover method, and useful in evaluating a single patient response to a short-acting agent (Guyatt *et al.* 1990). Nonrandomized comparative group designs and one-group noncomparative open designs lack the rigour of the randomized parallel, crossover and sequential trial designs. The use of a placebo prevents the outcome: drug $A =$ drug $B = 0$.

Patient selection
Patients are selected ideally from a single diagnostic group. Selection, however, implies that certain patients will be excluded, with the consequence that conclusions can be made only on patients with the characteristics chosen for the study. Patients tend to be a homogeneous group whose disease is considered responsive to treatment and whose compliance is high.

Calculation of sample size
This can be done from published standard formulae. Several factors, however, are important, especially: the trial design, the magnitude of type I and type II

errors, the variability within and between the patient groups, and the magnitude of the minimum difference (i.e. the delta) between the treatment groups and placebo controls. These complexities and standard formulae for calculating sample size are discussed in standard textbooks (Lee *et al.* 1973). The greatest difficulty is in defining the delta and standard deviation, the former often being arrived at by guesswork.

Randomization and stratification

Randomization is a statistical method of attempting to increase the probability that undefined variables of potential prognostic importance are evenly distributed between the study groups. There are, however, no guarantees that such undefined variables are evenly distributed. Stratification on, the other hand, does allow for defined variables to be equally distributed. The most important variable in determining the response to an analgesic drug is the severity of pain present at baseline. Patients with severe pain will respond dramatically to an anti-inflammatory analgesic, whereas patients with mild or moderate pain will respond only to a small degree (Lee *et al.* 1973).

Despite randomization and stratification important prognostic variables can be overlooked in statistical analysis. Two alternative methods of assigning patients to treatment groups have been described to overcome such difficulties. These are minimization (Taves 1974) and self-adjusting randomization (Nordle and Brantmark 1977). Clinicians tend to be in awe of statisticians, failing to realize that clinical common sense is still superior to any statistical manoeuvre.

Intervention

This term refers to the specific treatment in the study. Doses of a drug may be fixed or titrated, the latter more closely following clinical practice. Washout periods, especially prior to the start of trials with nonsteroidal anti-inflammatory analgesics, ensure that patients can respond to treatment.

Co-intervention

Co-intervention is administration of another treatment, which may interfere with the results of a trial. This treatment may take many forms, which may not be drugs (e.g. physiotherapy). Acetaminophen or paracetamol is a common co-intervention in trials of nonsteroidal anti-inflammatory drugs, and its consumption is often used as a surrogate measure of pain control.

Contamination

Contamination occurs in patients in a trial being given inappropriate medication.

Compliance

Compliance is the extent to which a patient adheres to a treatment protocol. The degree of noncompliance that is clinically important remains to be determined.

The development of electronic monitoring devices has revealed gross over-estimates of compliance as measured by patient report, either verbal or diary, returned tablet counts and measurement of drug concentrations or traces or a drug contaminant (e.g. phenobarbitone in blood or urine) (Urquhart 2000). Patients with continuous severe pain, as in rheumatoid arthritis, have been found to be extremely compliant in taking analgesics.

Statistical analysis

Essentially there are two approaches to analysis. In the first, all patients failing to complete the study are excluded from analysis. In the second approach, all patients entered in the study are included in the intention-to-treat analysis. The second approach is currently the preferred method (Sackett and Gent 1979).

Recently there has been debate regarding whether significance levels are appropriate in analysing data in clinical trials, and whether it would be preferable to use confidence levels and equivalence testing (Simon 1986). Perhaps of even greater importance in the analysis of clinical trial data is discussion of the clinical importance of the results (Chan et al. 2001). The difference between statistical significance and clinical importance must always be borne in mind, and there is a case for authors of clinical trials to discuss this in their reports (Clarke and Chalmers 1998; Docherty and Smith 1999).

Meta-analysis

Meta-analysis is the statistical combination of results from several studies to produce a single estimate of the effect of a treatment. Meta-analysis is liable to numerous biases at the level of both the individual trial and the dissemination of trial results. Meta-analyses have given contradictory conclusions (Egger et al. 2001) and conclusions different from those obtained by conventional reviews (Felson et al. 1990; Gotzsche et al. 1992; Bailer 1997; Gould 1996). One of the problems facing meta-analysis is that negative trials are frequently not published, and many trials are published in what has been termed the "grey zone" (i.e. only as summaries).

■ OUTCOME MEASURES

Rubor et tumor cum calor et dolor
> Celsus (53 BC–AD 7)

Et functio laesa
> Paul Ehrlich (1815–1915) (Galen c 129–200)

Et rigor
> EC Huskisson (1976)

It is a sobering thought that clinical therapeutic trials of antirheumatic drugs are still based on the cardinal features of inflammation (Beecher 1959).

Dolor or pain is the most important symptom in both noninflammatory and inflammatory joint disease, and is measured in terms of its relief (Beecher 1959).

Several methods have been devised for assessing joint tenderness in rheumatoid arthritis, all of which have their advocates, and recently one has been devised for osteoarthritis and for ankylosing spondylitis. Tumour is assessed by measurement of the circumference of the proximal interphalangeal joints in the hands and the interphalangeal joint of the thumb. Reduction in circumference is a measure of a drug's anti-inflammatory effect, but is relatively crude.

Colour can be measured by thermography, but is too complicated for general use. Rubor is never measured, as it occurs only in acute gouty and septic arthritis. Measurement of *functio laesa* was the principal outcome in the first reported controlled clinical trial by Thomas N Fraser in 1945 (Fraser 1945). Since then a large number of functional indices and health status instruments have been developed with their own devotees. Most of these were developed for assessing rheumatoid arthritis, but one which has now gained universal favour, the WOMAC, has been designed for special use in patients with osteoarthritis (Bellamy *et al.* 1998). Rigor is frequently measured in trials of antirheumatic drugs in patients with inflammatory joint disease. Severity of joint stiffness is preferred to duration, which depends on when the patient wakens.

The aggregation of a number of different endpoints, which may include results of laboratory tests such as the erythrocyte sedimentation rate, is frequently used to provide an overall composite index (see Table 1 for evaluation of the effect of disease-modifying antirheumatic drugs or DMARDs). However, although this procedure has much to commend it, the appropriate basis for the differential weighting of the individual components remains controversial.

Radiological scoring systems have been evolved to assess effects of drugs in preventing joint damage (Sharp 2000). These have been used especially in long-term trials of so-called DMARDs in rheumatoid arthritis. In should be noted, however, that there is a high inter-rater error in interpreting erosions even among skilled radiologists, and that fresh erosions may appear as others heal.

Whatever measure is used in clinical therapeutic trials it is important that the intraobserver variability be recorded, such as is the custom in laboratory tests.

■ EVIDENCE-BASED MEDICINE

Although the randomized placebo-controlled clinical trial is generally recognized as the "gold" standard for the assessment of drugs, and is the basis of evidence-based medicine (Heberden 1929/1994), it has to be appreciated that it also has "clay feet". This concept applies not only to general internal medicine, but also to its subspecialties, including rheumatology. However, as Downie and Macnaughton (2000) of Glasgow University have pointed out, judgement is integral to all activities in medical research. Furthermore, the treatment of patients requires not only evidence of drug efficacy, but also knowledge of drug chemistry, pharmacokinetics, drug–disease and drug–drug interactions and disease pathophysiology.

The major criticism of randomized clinical trials is that they deal with a narrow population of patients, who are not necessarily representative of the

Table 1 Evaluation of DMARD effect

ACR improvement criteria
- tender joint count*
- swollen joint count
- at least three of:
  - global disease activity—investigator
  - global disease activity—patient**
  - patient assessment of pain
  - physical disability score (e.g. HAQ)
  - acute phase reactant

ACR 20, ACR 50 and ACR 70 indicate 20%, 50% and 70% improvement in the above.

EULAR response criteria
Disease activity score (DAS) is derived using a nomogram which incorporates the following four measures:

- Ritchie articular index
- swollen joint count
- erythrocyte sedimentation rate (Westergren)
- general health score

DAS >2.8 is the usual level of activity for enrolment in DMARD studies. Interpretation of change in disease activity score from baseline evaluation of response:

>1.2 good
>0.6 moderate ≤1.2
≤0.6 nonresponders

Radiological assessment

Sharp method (scores erosions and joint space narrowing)
Larsen method (utilizes standardized films that illustrate progressive destructive disease)

*Extent of synovitis is measured by counting number of tender joints and number that are both swollen and tender.
**Patient opinion of disease activity measured on a 10 cm visual analogue scale. Anchor points at either end of the scale are "not active at all" and "extremely active".

general population. Patients at the extremes of life, women of child-bearing years, and those with other diseases are almost always excluded. The patients are therefore what Americans would describe as "squeaky clean", and as a consequence the results are not necessarily generalizable to "real world" patients.

Those who agree to participate in randomized controlled clinical trials differ from those who refuse to do so. Therapeutic trials are double-blind, but absent from most publications is information on how many patients were able to break the code. How double-blind is double-blind? And does it matter? In short-term trials on nonsteroidal anti-inflammatory analgesics breaking the code is perhaps of little importance but it probably does matter in long-term studies of disease-modifying antirheumatic agents.

It is generally not appreciated that side-effects, both mild and severe, potentiate analgesic effects (Max *et al.* 1998) and this is never addressed in publications on antirheumatic drug trials. Placebos are pharmacologically inert drugs or procedures that are prescribed with therapeutic intent. However, patients who are recruited for clinical therapeutic trials must be informed that they will receive an inert drug or sham treatment. As a consequence there are, strictly speaking, no placebo-controlled trials. Patients' preconceived preference on outcome is never considered, and may be of considerable importance in a study of a new "wonder" drug.

The major weakness of a randomized controlled clinical trial, and hence of evidence-based medicine, is that the degree of improvement deals with the average, not the individual patient. Average is not a reality: variation is the real reality (Gould 1996). Clinical therapeutic trials essentially test the *pharmacological effectiveness* of a drug, not its *therapeutic value*. They do not indicate how best an individual patient should be treated, which depends on both experience and clinical judgement.

The search for a more scientific basis for our therapeutic endeavours has a long history. James Lind (1716–1794), an Edinburgh graduate on board the British naval ship *Salisbury*, conducted the first controlled, but not double-blind, trial demonstrating the efficacy of citrus fruit in preventing and treating scurvy (Lind 1753). Lind in his treatise states, "I shall propose nothing merely dictated from theory, but shall confirm all by experience and facts, the surest and most unerring guides". Pierre Charles Alexandre Louis (1787–1872), working in Paris in the first half of the 19th century, can be considered the founder of quantitative medicine, averring that "without the aid of statistics nothing like real medicine is possible" (Louis 1835). If we were to accept the evidence of the innumerable properly controlled studies on the role of acid production in the pathogenesis of peptic ulcer we would continue to order alkali powders, milk drips and H_2 blockers to treat peptic ulcer. The recognition that peptic ulcer was due to *Helicobacter pylori* has revolutionized treatment, so that cure can be achieved after a single course of antimicrobial treatment (Peterson 1991). This major therapeutic advance was made not by a controlled clinical trial, but by questioning the role of the organism in the pathogenesis of peptic ulcer.

Prognosis

In assessing drug therapy it is important to keep in mind the natural history of the disease. This is particularly germane to the assessment of disease-modifying antirheumatic drugs and biologics in rheumatoid arthritis.

■ DRUG TOXICITY

Measurement of adverse drug reactions has received, in comparison to evaluation of efficacy, relatively little attention. Adverse rates differ on whether responses are volunteered or elicited. Most drugs are licensed after clinical trials in 3000 to 5000 patients, so that only common adverse reactions are identified. The rule of 3 is useful: if an adverse reaction occurs in 1 of 3 patients, then 3×3 (i.e. 9 patients will be required to be seen before it is 95% certain that the side-effect is recorded). If the reaction is 1 in 3000, or 1 in 5000, then 9000 and 15 000 patients respectively will require to be seen. Clearly if the adverse reaction is rare (i.e. 1 in 100 000 then some 300 000 will need to be seen before being 95% certain of identifying it).

Adverse drug reactions are of two types:

- More common, dose dependent and generally less severe.
- Idiosyncratic reactions, rarer and more likely to be serious.

A number of post-marketing reporting systems are in place in many countries. In the United Kingdom the Yellow Card Scheme of spontaneous reporting has had a number of successes despite its many weaknesses. The scheme is limited in that reactions are linked to a drug by association rather than by causation. Also, during the first two years of a new drug being on the market, numerous reactions are reported (the Weber effect), which rapidly fall off. The Yellow Card Scheme, and similar schemes, has the drawback that it lacks the denominator of the total number of prescriptions.

Pharmacoepidemiological studies including record-linkage systems can assess large numbers of patients with different diseases and of different gender and age, but to date these have not proved particularly helpful. Venning (1983) in a study of adverse reactions with 18 drugs in the United Kingdom noted that they were first identified in single anecdotal reports. The series of publications by O'Brien and Bagby (1985) on rare side-effects of antirheumatic drugs amply testify to the clinical awareness of individual physicians.

■ CO-MORBIDITY

Effective management of co-morbidity is a vital component of care of patients with rheumatoid arthritis and other inflammatory arthropathies. Particular attention should be paid to:

- Cardiovascular morbidity including hypertension and ischaemic heart disease
- Osteoporosis
- Anaemia
- Depression
- Increased risk of infection
- Other autoimmune conditions (e.g. thyroid disease).

■ OVERALL MANAGEMENT OF PATIENTS WITH INFLAMMATORY ARTHRITIS

In addition to pharmacological interventions detailed, the following should be remembered:

■ Involve the physiotherapist at all stages; dynamic exercise is of proven benefit.
■ Pay attention to home and working environments with the help of the occupational therapist.
■ Provide dietary and exercise advice.
■ Involve the social worker where necessary.
■ Encourage the patient to become involved in disease management. Education/self-help through programmes run by Arthritis Care may be valuable.

2 NSAIDs

N onsteroidal anti-inflammatory drugs

■ INTRODUCTION

An appraisal of the efficacy of nonsteroidal anti-inflammatory drugs (NSAIDs) in inflammatory arthritis requires some awareness of their development. It is noteworthy from the perspective of the contributors to this formulary that it was a Scottish physician, Thomas MacLagan, in 1874 who is credited for the use of salicin (the active principle of willow bark) as an antipyretic. Subsequently, the benefits of salicin in relieving the arthritic symptoms of rheumatic fever became apparent. Acetylsalicylic acid, the first NSAID, was synthesized in 1853. It was, however, not until 1967 that Boardman and Hart undertook the definitive clinical trial, a two-week crossover study to confirm the efficacy of high-dose aspirin in rheumatoid arthritis (RA): high-dose aspirin was equivalent to corticosteroids in reducing joint size and improving grip strength.

Subsequent development was driven by the need to develop an agent with an efficacy similar to that of high-dose aspirin but without the gastrointestinal (GI) side-effects, a goal that remains relevant today. The first of the many alternatives was mefenamic acid. Available NSAIDs now have only a tenuous structural similarity to aspirin. Despite this, both aspirin and NSAIDSs mediate their benefit and harm by cycloxygenase (COX) or prostaglandin synthetase inhibition (see Figure 1). The recognition of two isoforms—COX-1 (a housekeeping enzyme fundamental for efficient cellular functioning) and COX-2 (induced by inflammatory stimuli)—has led to the development of drugs that specifically inhibit COX-2 rather than COX-1.

NSAIDs are best considered as those with a short and long half-life. The previous chemical classifications of NSAIDs have no practical advantage. As some NSAIDs either selectively or specifically inhibit COX-2 this provides the basis for another useful classification (see Table 1 on commonly used NSAIDs).

■ BENEFITS

NSAIDs relieve the pain and stiffness typical of inflammatory arthritis as well as the cardinal signs of inflammation of calor, dolor, turgor and rubor. Efficacy is judged in terms of relief of pain and stiffness, joint swelling and tenderness. They have no effect on erythrocyte sedimentation rate (ESR), C-reactive protein (CRP) or radiological progression.

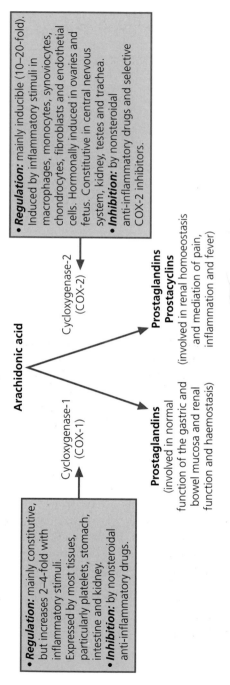

Figure 1 Action, regulation and inhibition of cycloxygenase-1 and cycloxygenase-2.

Table 1 Commonly used NSAIDs and maximum daily dose for RA

Drug	Maximum daily dose
Nonselective	
Diclofenac	150 mg
Flurbiprofen	200 mg
Ibuprofen	2400 mg
Indomethacin	150 mg
Ketoprofen	200 mg
Nabumetone	1500 mg
Naproxen	1000 mg
Sulindac	400 mg
COX-2 selective	
Etodolac	600 mg
Meloxicam	15 mg
Celecoxib	400 mg
Etoricoxib	90 mg
Rofecoxib	25 mg

Differences between NSAIDs

Although 24 agents are listed in the *British National Formulary*, in routine practice it is necessary to be familiar with only a few (see Table 1 on commonly prescribed NSAIDs). NSAIDs at equipotent doses in comparative studies show little difference in efficacy, but differences in response in individual patients is well recognized in clinical practice. This remains unexplained and may be due to pharmacodynamic rather than pharmacokinetic differences. There is no difference in efficacy between COX-1 and COX-2 in either selective or specific inhibitors.

Comparison of side-effects between COX-2-specific inhibitors and other NSAIDs reveals evidence of reduced GI toxicity but similar effects on the kidney and cardiovascular system. Initial studies suggest that COX-2-specific inhibitors are safe in patients with aspirin-induced asthma. Although celecoxib lists sulphonamide allergy as a contraindication, available data suggest an overall low incidence of hypersensitivity with celecoxib. However, occasional cases of hypersensitivity reaction including urticaria, angio-oedema and Stevens–Johnson syndrome have been described with both celecoxib and rofecoxib. A major benefit of the COX-2-specific inhibitors is that they do not interfere with platelet function and therefore can be used in situations where there is a bleeding problem, perioperatively or with anticoagulants.

■ RISKS

Although declining, the mortality from NSAIDs remains unacceptably high; one estimate puts it greater than that of acquired immune deficiency syndrome in the United States. Table 2 shows the recognized side-effects of NSAIDs and Table 3 the most frequent adverse reactions reported to the UK Committee for Safety of Medicines (CSM).

Table 2 Side-effects of nonselective NSAIDs	
Gastrointestinal (common)	Indigestion, ulceration, haemorrhage Small-bowel ulceration Stomatitis
Renal (common)	Transient rise in serum creatinine level Renal failure Oedema Interstitial nephritis Papillary necrosis Hyperkalaemia
Neurological (uncommon)	Headache Aseptic meningitis Dizziness Nausea
Pulmonary (rare)	Asthma Pulmonary oedema Pulmonary alveolitis
Dermatological (rare)	Erythema multiforme or variants (Stevens–Johnson syndrome and toxic epidermal necrolysis) Bullous eruptions Benign morbilliform eruptions Photosensitivity Fixed drug eruption Urticaria Pustular psoriasis
Haematological (rare)	Aplastic anaemia Red-cell aplasia Thrombocytopenia Haemolytic anaemia
Hepatic (rare)	Hepatitis Reye's syndrome
Systemic (rare)	Anaphylactoid reactions

Table 3 CSM notification of NSAID side-effects: 10 most common reports

Conventional NSAIDs		COX-2 selective	n (%)	
GI symptoms	11 483 (14%)	General	953	(12%)
Rashes	10 339 (13%)	GI symptoms and signs	533	(8%)
"General"	6651 (8%)	CVS symptoms and signs	533	(7%)
Upper GI perforation	4630 (6%)	Rashes	429	(6%)
CVS symptoms and signs	2672 (3%)	Upper GI perforation	252	(3%)
Gastrointestinal haemorrhage	2469 (3%)	Respiratory signs and symptoms	245	(3%)
Urticaria	2385 (3%)	Miscellaneous skin and tissue disease	218	(3%)
Angio-oedema	1936 (2%)	Headache	195	(3%)
Miscellaneous skin and tissue disease	1905 (2%)	Angio-oedema	156	(2%)
Headache	1749 (2%)	Gastrointestinal haemorrhages	126	(2%)
Of total	**82 077**	**Of total**	**7628**	

GI, gastrointestinal; CVS, cardiovascular system.

Gastrointestinal

NSAID damage can occur throughout the GI tract. Side-effects include:

- Dyspepsia, heartburn, nausea/vomiting, abdominal pain (15–40%)
- Endoscopic mucosal lesions (40%)
- Serious GI complications (e.g. perforation or bleeding) (1.5%/year)

Symptoms correlate poorly with endoscopic findings and are often absent prior to major complications. Endoscopic gastric ulcers are approximately ten times more common than duodenal ulcers. It is, however, the complications of gastro-duodenal ulceration that are more important. Although the incidence of gastroduodenal complications may appear low, NSAIDs are so widely used that there is a significant impact in the at-risk population. Risk of complications is highest in the elderly woman with a history of peptic ulcer and cardiac disease (18%).

The risk of NSAID ulcer complications increases directly with:

- Age, being highest in those over 65 years
- A history of peptic ulceration
- Co-morbidity (e.g. cardiac disease)
- Higher NSAID dose
- The use of two NSAIDs (including aspirin for cardiovascular disease prophylaxis)
- Concomitant corticosteroid and anticoagulant use
- Co-existing *Helicobacter pylori* infection

The most frequent serious complication is bleeding. There is a hierarchy of risk for GI bleeding with nonselective NSAIDs.

Advice to minimize GI side-effects of NSAIDs
- Start at lowest recommended dose
- Do not use more than one NSAID concomitantly
- Combinations of non-aspirin NSAID and low-dose aspirin may be associated with increased risk
- Use for shortest duration of time (effective DMARD use should reduce NSAID requirements)
- Be aware that azapropazone and piroxicam have high GI risk profiles
- Consider COX-2 selective agent
- Consider use of gastroprotective agent

■ GI PROTECTIVE AGENTS

- Misoprostol
- Proton pump inhibitors
- H_2 antagonists

Symptoms

H_2 antagonists may be a reasonable option in treating dyspepsia in those at low risk of complications. Proton pump inhibitors were effective in providing symptom relief in comparative studies with misoprostol, which is often not well tolerated in doses to prevent complications. There was no difference in the incidence of symptoms between conventional NSAIDs and either selective or specific COX-2 inhibitors.

Ulcers

Conventional doses of H_2 blockers reduce the frequency of duodenal but not gastric ulcers. Higher doses also reduce the incidence of gastric ulcers. Proton pump inhibitors are superior to misoprostol in prevention of duodenal ulcers, but efficacy is similar for gastric ulcers. COX-2-specific inhibitors significantly reduce the incidence of endoscopic ulceration.

Ulcer-related complications

Only misoprostol prevents perforation and gastric outlet obstruction. The evidence for prevention of GI bleeding is suggestive but not definitive for misoprostol. There are no outcome studies for high-dose H_2 blockers or proton pump inhibitors. Longer-term results from the CLASS study suggest that the protective effect of celecoxib (in the absence of concomitant aspirin) on the GI tract is lost by 12 months, although other studies (e.g. VIGOR), suggest a more sustained response.

Relevance of *Helicobacter pylori*

Individual studies on the relative contribution of *H. pylori* in the pathogenesis of NSAID-induced gastroduodenal ulceration have provided conflicting results. A recent meta-analysis of published studies (only 25 of 463 publications were judged to be of rigorous enough methodology to be included) showed that both risk factors had a synergistic effect, increasing the risk of peptic ulceration 20-fold compared to either risk factor alone. It was not possible to calculate the relative contributions of each in gastric and duodenal ulceration, as most studies did not distinguish between the two. In those that did, there was a stronger association between *H. pylori* and duodenal ulcers and NSAIDs with gastric ulcers. The presence of both also increased the risk of GI bleeding. The role of *H. pylori* in the context of peptic ulcer-related complications with a specific COX-2 inhibitor has not been tested.

Should *H. pylori* status therefore be sought and eradication therapy undertaken in all patients requiring long-term NSAID treatment? The results of one recent controlled trial suggest that there may be an advantage in those with dyspepsia or history of an ulcer.

A pragmatic eradication policy may be:

- In patients with a history of peptic ulcer disease or persistent dyspepsia requiring long-term NSAID treatment.
- If a patient on NSAID therapy develops an ulcer with evidence of infection.

■ RISKS OF NSAIDs OTHER THAN GI SYMPTOMS

Hypertension

NSAIDs increase supine blood pressure by a mean of 5 mmHg. The increase may be greater in some hypertensive patients, particularly those on a beta blocker or a diuretic. The long-term consequences of such a persistent rise in blood pressure are not known, but may be one explanation for the increased cardiovascular mortality observed in RA. There is some evidence that calcium channel blockers may be preferable in treating hypertensive patients requiring NSAID treatment.

Heart failure

NSAID-induced systemic vasoconstriction significantly increases the risk of deterioration in patients with pre-existing heart failure; patients with hyponatraemia are at greatest risk.

Thrombosis

Concern regarding the potential prothrombotic effects of specific COX-2 inhibitors initially arose due to case reports and was further highlighted in the VIGOR study. This study was designed to evaluate the benefit of rofecoxib over naproxen in RA patients with regard to gastroduodenal ulcer complications. An early finding that became more apparent as the study progressed was the higher incidence of thrombotic events in rofecoxib patients. Three explanations have been offered:

1. Naproxen has a cardioprotective effect similar to that of aspirin. Controversy surrounds the cardioprotective effects of NSAIDs, one view being that they may be deleterious.
2. Rofecoxib is pro-thrombotic. This observation from the VIGOR study is not supported by data from other studies. Furthermore, the VIGOR study was neither designed nor powered to establish a pro-thrombotic tendency.
3. The results occurred by chance.

A useful guidance if a COX-2 agent is chosen in a patient with cardiovascular risk factors is to administer aspirin and, if risk factors for GI toxicity are present, to consider the use of a proton pump inhibitor. In those with a history of peptic ulceration, in particular duodenal ulcers, *H. pylori* eradication should be considered.

Renal

NSAID-induced renal failure can arise owing to haemodynamic effects or secondary to interstitial nephritis. Renal prostaglandins have an important role in maintaining renal perfusion in the presence of glomerular disease, renal impairment or disorders in which secretion of the vasoconstrictor angiotensin II is increased. Inhibition in these circumstances leads to ischaemia and a reduction in glomerular filtration rate. These effects can occur with all NSAIDs including the specific COX-2 inhibitors, although there is some evidence that sulindac has less of an effect on renal prostaglandin synthesis. Interstitial inflammation can occur with any NSAID, is presumed to be an idiosyncratic reaction, and may be associated with a minimal-change glomerulonephritis.

It is unresolved whether long-term use of NSAIDs results in papillary necrosis and hence analgesic nephropathy.

Hepatitis

Increases in transaminase levels are common with NSAID use; in most instances elevations are mild and resolve on drug withdrawal. The risk is higher in patients with RA compared to those with osteoarthritis and in particular with sulindac and diclofenac. With both it is thought to be an idiosyncratic reaction. In those patients receiving long-term NSAID treatment, liver function tests should be carried out within the first three months of initiating treatment.

Hypersensitivity reactions

Urticaria, angio-oedema and bronchospasm due to aspirin as well as other NSAIDs can occur together or as individual complications. Rechallenge with another NSAID is not advised but if absolutely necessary can be undertaken in a controlled environment, as most reactions occur within 30 minutes of ingestion. Interactions are shown in Table 4.

Table 4 Interactions with NSAIDs

Drug combination*	Potential result
Anticoagulants/oxphenbutazone Phenylbutazone	Markedly potentiate effect of warfarin
Anticoagulants/all NSAIDs	Increased risk of bleeding due to additive effects of gastric mucosal damage and inhibition of platelet function
Beta blockers, vasodilators†/NSAIDs to varying degrees‡	Loss of hypotensive and diuretic effects
Methotrexate/NSAIDs	Decreased renal clearance of methotrexate—particularly with high doses of methotrexate
Lithium/NSAIDs	Increased plasma lithium concentrations
Antacid agents/salicylates	Decreased plasma salicylate concentrations
Antacid agents/NSAIDs (other than salicylates)	Slowing of absorption of some NSAIDs
Sulfonylurea/oxphenbutazone Phenylbutazone	Inhibition of sulfonylurea metabolism and risk of hypoglycaemia
Corticosteroids/salicylates	Decreased plasma salicylate concentrations
Phenytoin/phenylbutazone	Increased plasma phenytoin concentrations causing toxicity

*Drug interactions in the first column have the potential to be clinically significant.
†Hydralazine, prazosin, captopril.
‡Less with sulindac.

3 DMARDs

There is abundant evidence that early disease-modifying antirheumatic drug (DMARD) therapy in rheumatoid arthritis (RA) improves clinical and laboratory parameters five years after initiation of therapy. Delayed introduction of DMARDs is associated with a less favourable outcome in terms of morbidity and mortality. There are clear analogies with tight control of hypertension and diabetes: early and sustained suppression of disease confers long-term advantages.

Early introduction of DMARDs is of particular importance in patients who are seropositive for rheumatoid factor (RF), have high inflammatory markers such as erythrocyte sedimentation rate (ESR) or C-reactive protein (CRP), or who have many synovitic joints at presentation.

Sustained suppression of synovitis and the acute-phase response is associated with better functional outcome, less erosive damage to joints, reduced requirements for joint replacement surgery and a reduction in the "lost years" (i.e. an improvement in premature mortality associated with RA).

The choice of initial DMARD is dictated by patient and physician, once clinical features or co-morbidities have been taken into consideration.

Hydroxychloroquine may be useful where doubt exists about possible connective tissue disease onset or overlap of connective tissue disease with inflammatory arthritis.

Most rheumatologists would now choose either sulphasalazine or methotrexate as their initial DMARD for RA, switching to the other or adding another if the effect is suboptimal.

Intramuscular (IM) gold, leflunomide, D-penicillamine or azathioprine are other available options. Auranofin and cyclosporin are less often used, the former because of inefficiency, the latter because of renal toxicity.

3 DMARDs

HYDROXYCHLOROQUINE

> **KEY INDICATIONS**
> - Rheumatoid arthritis
> - Systemic lupus erythematosus

■ INTRODUCTION

Antimalarials have been used to treat rheumatoid arthritis (RA) since the late 1950s. The precise rationale for their use remains uncertain. Early studies (Rinehart *et al.* 1957; Cohen and Calkins 1958; Kersley and Palin 1959) used chloroquine with benefit in RA. Later analyses, albeit small, used hydroxychloroquine and showed efficacy comparable to that of placebo and a reduced corticosteroid requirement (Mainland and Sutcliffe 1962) or analgesic dose (Hamilton and Scott 1962). A later uncontrolled study found that 12% of RA patients improved to the point of possible remission (Adams *et al.* 1983). A dose-ranging study failed to show a numerical benefit for use at 400 mg/day as compared to 200 mg/day (Pavelka *et al.* 1989). All studies demonstrate a low toxicity profile for hydroxychloroquine and it is perhaps this that remains an attraction for its continued use.

■ PHARMACOLOGY

Absorption of hydroxychloroquine varies from 30% to 100%; 40% is bound to plasma proteins and there is no therapeutic range established. The half-life of antimalarials, including hydroxychloroquine, is in the order of 40 days. It is estimated that the time for steadystate concentrations to be attained is about six months (Tett 1993). Hydroxychloroquine is metabolized primarily to oxidative byproducts that have high renal clearances. A direct relationship between levels of desethylhydroxychloroquine (one of these metabolites) and efficacy suggests that it may not be hydroxychloroquine itself that is efficacious (Munster *et al.* 2002). In contrast, gastrointestinal side-effects were more common in patients with higher hydroxychloroquine levels, implying a causative relationship with the parent compound.

■ BENEFIT

Four randomized controlled studies have compared hydroxychloroquine at a dose of 400 mg/day to placebo (Davis *et al.* 1991; Clarke *et al.* 1993; Blackburn *et al.* 1995; Esdaile *et al.* 1995). None provides enough information to calculate ACR or Paulus responses to demonstrate any change in these parameters, rather they analysed individual criteria for improvement.

The results of the Hydroxychloroquine in Early Rheumatoid Arthritis (HERA) study (Esdaile *et al.* 1995) are typical of the response expected with hydroxychloroquine (see Figure 1). There was an improvement on composite score including painful and swollen joints, grip strength and duration of early morning stiffness (p < 0.0004), pain index (p < 0.007) and the combination of

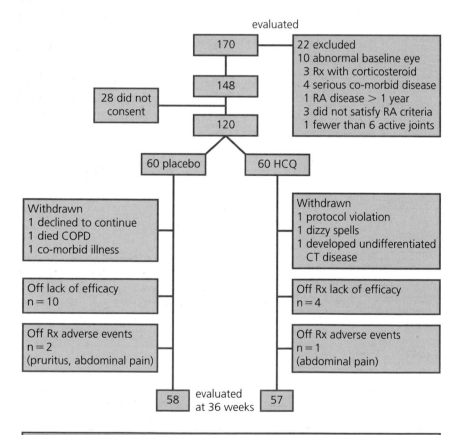

Figure 1 Hydroxychloroquine (HCQ) in early RA in the HERA study (36 weeks). COPD, chronic obstructive pulmonary disease.

disability scores from a variety of self-assessment questionnaires ($p < 0.02$). In addition there was a small improvement in the hydroxychloroquine group using the global index of patients and assessors ($p < 0.03$).

Meta-analysis (Suarez-Almazor *et al.* 2000) clearly shows an improvement in a basket of parameters including tender joints, swollen joints and erythrocyte sedimentation rate (ESR) but not pain, global assessments or radiological scores, and confirms fewer withdrawals in the treatment groups due to lack of efficacy.

A three-year follow-up of the HERA study cohort after the first phase of the study (Tsakonas *et al.* 2000) showed that the initial placebo group always had worse pain index, functional index and sense of global well-being, adding to the argument for mandatory early DMARD therapy in RA.

The relative slow onset of efficacy and low toxicity of conventional hydroxy-chloroquine treatment (reviewed in Suarez-Almazor *et al.* 2000) has led to the suggestion that an initial high dose could be more effective in early treatment. In a dose-loading study using Paulus criteria there was a trend towards a better response in those receiving higher doses for the first six weeks at the expense of a higher toxicity profile (see Table 1).

Unfortunately, this study was under-powered, but nevertheless this trend was observed ($p = 0.052$), and when comparing the individual components of the Paulus criteria numerical superiority was with the higher doses (Furst *et al.* 1999).

■ COMPARISON STUDIES WITH OTHER DMARDs

Several studies have compared hydroxychloroquine with other DMARDs. All demonstrated that hydroxychloroquine was less effective than other DMARDS, but had a lower toxicity profile.

Bunch *et al.* (1984) compared hydroxychloroquine with D-penicillamine in a controlled study. In both groups there was an improvement from baseline in a variety of parameters favouring penicillamine. In a comparison between aura-nofin and hydroxychloroquine there were only minor differences in clinical efficacy (Bird *et al.* 1984). The low toxicity profile was confirmed in both studies. A five-year analysis found that 5% of hydroxychloroquine-treated patients stopped

Table 1 Comparison of response to increasing doses of hydroxychloroquine in rheumatoid arthritis (Furst *et al.* 1999)

Dose mg/day	Responders (Paulus criteria) (%)	Terminated therapy (%)
400	48	4
800	58	18
1200	64	27

therapy because of side-effects whereas ~15% stopped auranofin and penicillamine for these reasons (Jessop *et al.* 1998).

In a comparative study of hydroxychloroquine and sulphasalazine using conventional doses over 48 weeks Nuver-Zwart *et al.* (1989) found numerical superiority in all parameters in the sulphasalazine group with sustained improvement in pain score, grip strength, swollen joints and ESR, C-reactive protein (CRP) and levels of immunoglobulins. Although these improved statistically from respective baseline results, there was no difference when the two groups were compared together. This was confirmed by a subsequent analysis using smaller doses of hydroxychloroquine (Faarvang *et al.* 1993). In both studies the improvement was more rapid with sulphasalazine, and more patients dropped out because of lack of efficacy in the hydroxychloroquine group, in keeping with the later five-year comparison (Jessop *et al.* 1998). However, van der Heijde *et al.* (1989) showed, in a sulphasalazine/hydroxychloroquine comparison, that those in the sulphasalazine group developed fewer new erosions, and those with X-ray damage already present showed a slower deterioration than those in the hydroxychloroquine group. This indicates that sulphasalazine is more effective than hydroxychloroquine at reducing joint damage, but does not answer the question of hydroxychloroquine versus placebo.

In a more recent comparison, minocycline was found to be superior to hydroxychloroquine in early RA (see the section on Minocycline and Table 2).

■ POSSIBLE EFFECT ON CARDIOVASCULAR CO-MORBIDITY

In a comparative study of hydroxychloroquine and intramuscular (IM) gold on lipid profiles in RA patients there was a comparable fall in ESR, CRP and articular index (Munro *et al.* 1997) (similar to that of DMARDs in the Jessop trial, 1998). However, this analysis did show that hydroxychloroquine improved the lipid profile in RA to an extent equivalent to that in patients with systemic lupus erythematosus (SLE) (Petri *et al.* 1994).

Table 2 Comparison of response to hydroxychloroquine and minocycline in rheumatoid arthritis (O'Dell 2001)

n	Hydroxychloroquine	Minocycline	p Value
ACR 20	43%	67%	0.06
ACR 50	33%	60%	0.04
ACR 70	27%	43%	0.14
Pred dose (mg)	3.2	0.8	<0.01

■ TOXICITY

Nonocular toxicity

Hydroxychloroquine is regarded as a relatively nontoxic drug in comparison to other DMARDs. However, all the above studies show risks of the following adverse events:

- Gastrointestinal (10–34%).
- Neurological (5–13%).
- Dermatological (3–10%) problems associated with its use, but rarely so severe as to lead to treatment termination.
- In a result of two meta-analyses, only 2.3% stopped treatment because of dermatological side-effects (3.3% with gastrointestinal problems and 1% with neurological toxicity).

Table 3   Toxicity of hydroxychloroquine

	Symptoms	Findings	Management
Mucocutaneous	Pruritus Urticarial rashes Stomatitis	Rare	Withdraw
Gastrointestinal	Anorexia Nausea Vomiting Abdominal pain Diarrhoea	Uncommon	↓dose
CNS	Headache Dizziness Tinnitus	Uncommon	↓dose
Eyes	Blurred vision (resolves on continued therapy) Accommodation problems (resolves on continued therapy) Photophobia Retinal damage	Uncommon	May continue ↓dose STOP drug
Pregnancy	Crosses placenta, theoretically hazardous Reputed increase in retinal toxicity Cochlear toxicity Cardiorespiratory failure can occur	Very rare	Discontinue in pregnancy

■ In comparison with other DMARDs, significant liver and renal damage and bone marrow suppression were not reported with hydroxychloroquine use. Symptoms of myasthenia gravis might deteriorate during hydroxychloroquine treatment.

Ocular toxicity

The major concern with antimalarial use is that of ocular toxicity. Blurred vision occurs in up to 3% of patients (usually due to corneal deposits), and is reversible. However, retinal deposition of hydroxychloroquine is a concern because this is more common in older patients on longer-term treatment, is irreversible and may worsen with time (Marks and Power 1979; Finbloom et al. 1985). Analysis of results of visual screening of large numbers of patients taking hydroxychloroquine in various studies showed similar results to those of Grierson (1997). In this study of 758 patients, 12 developed visual disturbances with 10 having Amsler chart defects (none related to retinal toxicity) and seven developing temporary corneal deposits which improved on stopping treatment. Mavrikakis et al. (1996) reported retinal lesions in two of 58 patients on hydroxychloroquine for more than 6 years.

This has led to a review of the data (Silman and Shipley 1997) and papers (Fielder et al. 1998 and Canadian Consensus Conference 2000) that set out guidelines for screening in rheumatology clinics (see Table 4) and when to refer patients for more detailed examination by ophthalmologists.

Pregnancy and lactation

Hydroxychloroquine crosses the placenta and hence poses a theoretical risk. The British National Formulary suggests avoiding its use in pregnancy and lactation. Two studies have reported no teratogenicity following exposure to anti-malarials during early pregnancy; both analyses, although reassuring, were small (Parke 1988; Levey et al. 1991). Reports of an increased risk of cochlear damage following exposure to chloroquine have led to suggestions that hydroxychloroquine should not be used for this reason (ABPI Datasheet compendium 2000–2001).

Table 4   Ophthalmological screening and advice on referral (guidelines modified from the Royal College of Ophthalmologists recommendations)

Baseline screening
Ask about uncorrectable visual impairment
Record near visual acuity (with glasses if necessary) for both eyes using reading chart
If any impairment present then refer to optician, who would refer on if required

Annual evaluation
The recommended dose should not exceed 6.5 mg/kg/day
Review visual symptoms and acuity, and assess for blurred vision using reading chart

Referral to ophthalmologist
Visual impairment or eye disease at baseline
Change in acuity or blurred vision developing on treatment
When hydroxychloroquine is not licensed (e.g. childhood)

DRUG INTERACTIONS

- Cimetidine may increase the plasma concentration of hydroxychloroquine
- Antacids may impair absorption
- Avoid concurrent use with amiodarone (↑risk of ventricular arrhythmia)
- Possible reduction in plasma concentration of digoxin
- Increased concentration of cyclosporin

SUMMARY OF EFFICACY

- Hydroxychloroquine is effective in patients with rheumatoid arthritis when compared to placebo. Efficacy is demonstrated in 60–80% of patients over six months' treatment.
- Clinical benefit includes functional assessment, joint count, pain, grip strength, morning stiffness, patient and observer assessment, ESR and haemoglobin.
- When compared to other DMARDs, hydroxychloroquine has a slower onset of benefit. It is not as effective as sulphasalazine or penicillamine.
- However, lower toxicity profile and limited requirement for blood monitoring make it a useful option for RA treatment. The low toxicity profile, low costs and improvement in lipid profile renders hydroxychloroquine a useful DMARD.
- It is likely to be a frequent component of combination therapy for RA in the future.
- It is particularly useful in early inflammatory arthritis where the diagnosis (?connective tissue disease, ?RA) is not yet certain.

KEY REFERENCES

- Suarez-Almazor et al. 2001

- van der Heijde et al. 1989

- O'Dell et al. 2001

- Munro et al. 1997

- Grierson 1997

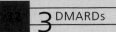

■ HYDROXYCHLOROQUINE—GP INFORMATION

Effect
Hydroxychloroquine is a mild second-line agent used for treatment of inflammatory arthritis and for skin and joint symptoms in connective tissue diseases. It may take 12–24 weeks before an effect is seen in inflammatory arthritis.

Prescribing
The recommended dose should not exceed 6.5 mg per kg per day. Starting dosage:

Patient weight	Dose
> 62 kg	400 mg per day
< 62 kg	200/400 mg alternate days
> 31 kg	200 mg per day

The dose may be reduced to 200 mg daily and below that, provided an adequate clinical response is achieved. It is recommended that treatment should be reviewed regularly after two years.

Monitoring
The patient should usually have baseline eye assessment. Record and document new visual acuity using a standard reading chart. Repeat annually. Patients should be advised to stop hydroxychloroquine if serious visual symptoms are experienced. Regular reviews by ophthalmologists are no longer necessary; blood and urine checks are not required.

Contraindications
■ Pregnancy and breast feeding are relative contraindications.
■ Dose should be reduced in renal impairment.
■ Antacids may impair absorption—take 30–60 minutes after hydroxychloroquine.

Adverse effects and management
Skin rashes	
Nausea	
Diarrhoea	May settle on reduced dose
Headache	Usually settles on reduced dose
Retinal deposits	The risk of maculopathy is negligible within two years of starting treatment
Corneal deposits	Usually reversible

3 DMARDs

SULPHASALAZINE

KEY INDICATIONS

- Rheumatoid arthritis
- Juvenile chronic arthritis
- Psoriatic arthritis
- Seronegative spondarthropathies including reactive arthritis

---

INTRODUCTION

Sulphasalazine (SASP) is a versatile drug in the treatment of inflammatory arthritis. It is an effective disease-modifying antirheumatic drug (DMARD) in rheumatoid arthritis (RA) and often the DMARD of first choice. It is also useful in psoriatic arthritis, in the seronegative spondarthropathies and in juvenile arthritis. The majority of side-effects occur early, and most reverse completely on cessation of therapy. Frequent monitoring, therefore, is necessary only in the first six months. No cumulative or unexpected long-term toxicity is known.

PHARMACOLOGY

SASP (salicyl azosulphapyridine) is a combination of sulphapyridine and 5-aminosalicylic acid linked by a diazo bond. Most reaches the colon intact where intestinal bacteria cleave the azo bond. The sulphapyridine moiety is rapidly absorbed. Plasma levels peak 3–6 hours after ingestion. It is widely distributed; synovial fluid concentrations are comparable to those in the serum. Before being excreted in the urine it undergoes acetylation and hydroxylation in the liver. In contrast, 5-aminosalicylic acid is poorly absorbed; most is excreted in the faeces. There is no evidence of a systemic anti-inflammatory response. Little of the intact SASP molecule is absorbed.

EFFICACY OF SASP IN THE TREATMENT OF RA

For many rheumatologists SASP is an anchor drug in RA. It is frequently used as the first DMARD *(widely used in Europe; 98% of Canadian rheumatologists prescribe SASP)*. Alternatives are methotrexate or leflunomide, both have a similar efficacy to SASP. Hydroxychloroquine is less effective.
Specific advantages include:

- A similar benefit in both seropositive and seronegative RA
- No dose adjustment is required for age or impaired renal function
- It is relatively inexpensive
- Frequent blood monitoring is required only in the first six months and thereafter every three months
- There is no cumulative toxicity and no adverse events are known with long-term treatment
- It is not known to be teratogenic, but is excreted in breast milk

EVIDENCE FOR BENEFIT IN RA

Table 1 shows the evidence for the clinical benefit of mono-therapy
Table 2 shows the two major meta-analyses
Table 3 shows the evidence for radiological outcomes in SASP
Table 4 shows the available information from long-term studies

■ COMPARATIVE STUDIES

SASP monotherapy

Between 1983 and 2000 ten randomized studies compared SASP with placebo and/or another DMARD (Figure 1). In the six that included a placebo group, significant benefit with SASP on clinical and laboratory parameters indicative of disease-modifying activity was noted. The expected improvement in duration of morning stiffness is 75%, Ritchie articular index, swollen joint count, tender joint count and erythrocyte sedimentation rate (ESR) is 50%. This usually occurs at 6–10 weeks of therapy. In comparison with intramuscular (IM) gold (sodium aurothiomalate), penicillamine, or leflunomide, there is a similar efficacy. Approximately two out of three patients will continue on treatment at one year. The ACR 20 and 50 responses are shown in Table 1.

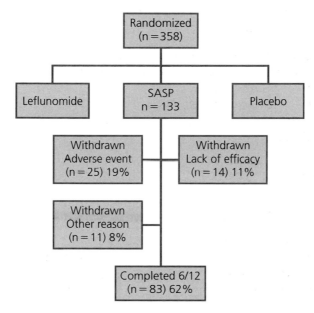

Figure 1 SASP Consort Diagram. From Smolen *et al.* 1999.

SASP has a greater magnitude of clinical benefit than hydroxychloroquine or auranofin and a more prompt response. Meta-analyses of SASP monotherapy confirm the equivalent clinical benefit of SASP, IM gold, D-penicillamine and methotrexate (Felson *et al.* 1990, 1992) with some evidence that patients remain longer on methotrexate and slightly more withdrawals for inefficacy than IM gold.

Radiology
SASP reduces the progression of radiological damage in RA. An early comparison of patients on SASP with those who persistently refused DMARDs showed less damage in SASP patients. This has been confirmed in a placebo-controlled study in which 17% of the placebo group showed progression of erosions compared to 5% of SASP- and 3% of leflunomide-treated patients over six months. There was no statistical difference between the SASP and leflunomide groups. The benefit of SASP on X-rays is greater than that of hydroxychloroquine (van der Heijole *et al.* 1989).

Long-term clinical efficacy results
Improvements in clinical and laboratory variables of disease activity is sustained over 5–10 years.

Table 1   Sulphasalazine in RA: comparative studies (randomized monotherapy)

Reference	n	Comparative drugs	Study design/disease duration	Duration of follow-up (months)	Outcome efficacy	Outcome toxicity	Conclusion/ comment
Pullar et al. 1983	90	SASP/IM gold/ placebo	Randomized, GST open, SASP/placebo-blind (6–9 year disease duration)	6	Significant clinical and laboratory benefit from SASP and gold Placebo: no benefit	Major SASP toxicity nausea and vomiting	SASP effective DMARD
Neuman et al. 1983	63	SASP/ D-penicillamine	Randomized open	4	SASP effective, equivalent to D-penicillamine	No major SASP side-effects. Nausea most common	SASP effective and safe
Pinals et al. 1986	86	SASP/placebo	Radomized controlled 6 year disease duration	4	Significantly more improvement in clinical and laboratory variables during SASP	28% withdrew during SASP. Side-effects not life-threatening. Reversed rapidly	Suppression of rheumatoid synovitis may be induced by SASP
Williams et al. 1988	186	SASP/IM gold/ placebo	Randomized controlled (4–7 year disease duration)	9	SASP similar in efficacy to injectable gold	SASP better tolerated than injectable gold	Greater placebo response than in previous studies
Nuver-Zwart et al. 1989	60	SASP/hydroxychloroquine	Radomized controlled (early disease <1.0 year)	12	Onset of response earlier with SASP. Lack of efficacy Withdrawals more with HCQ	Adverse reaction most common cause withdrawal of SASP. One agranulocytosis. All reversed completely	Earlier effect of SASP

Capell et al. 1990	200	SASP d-penicillamine	Radomized open (disease duration 7 years)	24	Majority of patients showed significant improvement in most parameters. 51% on Rx at 2 years SASP≡D-penicillamine	All side-effects reversed. Nausea responded to dose reduction on Rx with prochlorperazine in majority	No clinically relevant difference demonstrated between the 2 drugs
Australian Multicentre Group 1992	150	SASP/placebo	Randomized controlled early disease	6	Significant improvement with SASP cf placebo	Common side-effects rashes, abdominal LFTs, and GIT upset. All reversed	Demonstrated efficacy Of SASP in early RA
Hannonen et al. 1993	80	SASP/placebo	Radomized controlled early disease (4–6 months)	12	SASP superior to placebo	Few side-effects (5 on SASP). All reversed	SASP effective in treatment of RA and onset of action is rapid
Porter et al. 1992	200	SASP/auranofin	Radomized open (disease duration 9 years)	12	SASP onset of benefit more rapid. 63% on Rx at 1 year	Fewer side-effects in SASP group. Prompt recovery on withdrawal of Rx	SASP faster, possibly greater effect, with no increased toxicity
Smolen et al. 1999	358	SASP/leflunomide/ placebo	Radomized controlled ITT (mean disease duration 7 years)	6	ACR 20 56% SASP 55% LEF 29% placebo ACR 50 30% SASP 33% LEF 14% placebo SASP+LEFL ≡ superior to Placebo	2 SASP agranulocytosis reversed on withdrawal. Side-effects as expected	Similar response to leflunomide

Table 2 Meta-analysis of studies including sulphasalazine in RA

Reference	n studies/patients	Therapies	Duration	Outcome efficacy	Outcome toxicity	Verdict
Felson et al. 1990	66/117 Rx groups	SASP, MTX, GST, open, aur, antimalarials, placebo		Equivalent between SASP, GST, open and MTX	SASP < GST	
Felson et al. 1992	Updated 1990 Meta-analysis	As above				SASP relatively high potency and Only modest Toxicity
Weinblatt et al. 1999	15 studies	552 placebo, HCQ, open, GST	36 weeks	Compared to placebo SASP → improvement in ESR, VAS pain, AI, painful joints, Patient global. More withdrawals For inefficacy than GST	Fewer adverse effects than GST. More toxicity than placebo	More patients completed Rx with SASP, cf GST
Maetzel et al. 2000	110 studies	142 Rx arms MTX 48 GST 56 SASP 22 HCQ 16	24–60 months	Withdrawals for lack of efficacy MTX 25% GST 27% SASP 47%	Toxicity withdrawals MTX 35% GST 64% SASP 52%	36% on MTX 23% on GST 22% on SASP at 60 months

Table 3 Radiological damage as outcome measure in RA sulphasalazine studies

Reference	n	Comparative drugs	Study design	X-ray method	Outcome radiological scores	Conclusion
Pullar et al. 1987	51	"Placebo" (group who had refused DMARD over 2 years)	Cross-sectional 24 months	Modification of Sharp method	Median + 95% confidence intervals 0–1 year 1–2 years +4 +1 (+1 to +7) (-2 to +4)	Slowing of radiological progression in second year of therapy. Less deterioration than in patients who refused DMARD
van der Heijde et al. 1989	60	SASP/HCQ	Randomized double-blind over 12 months	Modified Sharp (hands). Erosions and joint space narrowing (feet)	Median erosion score Wk 0 24 48 SASP 1 2.5 5 HCQ 1 10 16	Statistically significant reduction in radiographic progression in SASP compared with HCQ
Sharp et al. 2000	358	SASP/LEF/ placebo	Randomized double-blind 6 months (continued to 12 months for active)	Modified Sharp method. Erosions and joint space narrowing	% of patients with radiographic progression SASP 5% LEF 3% Placebo 17%	SASP and LEF resulted in statistically significantly less radiological progression compared with placebo at 6 months

Table 4 Long-term studies of sulphasalazine in RA (5–12 years)

Reference	n	Comparative drugs	Duration of follow-up	Study design	Outcome efficacy	Outcome toxicity	Conclusion
Situnyake et al. 1990	891	SASP (315) IM gold (203) D-penicillamine (163)	5 years	Observational Not randomized	33% discontinued Rx because of inefficacy	No data presented	Improvements in SASP group maintained for 5 years (20% good response)
Jones et al. 1991	86	SASP (86)	5 years	Observational (prospective)	22% on Rx at 5 years 23% off Rx because of inefficacy	28% off Rx because of side-effect. Most adverse events in first 3 months. All reversible	Consider pessimistic reports of low continuation of DMARDs unfounded
Porter et al. 1994	675	SASP (222) IM gold (295) D-penicillamine (158)	5 years	Collected analysis of patients enrolled in prospective randomized studies in one unit	26% on Rx at 5 years with SASP 28% off Rx because of lack of loss of effect (cf 9% gold, 18% D-penicillamine)	33% off Rx SASP because of side-effect. All reversible (cf 45% gold, 42% D-penicillamine)	Good control of disease activity and improved function in 30% of RA patients. Rx with SASP/IM gold/D-penicillamine
van Riel et al. 1995	175	SASP (130) HCQ (45)	5 years	Prospective cohort study	35% on Rx at 5 years 9% in remission	Adverse reactions mainly in first 3 months. 20% off Rx because of toxicity. All reversible	Statistically significant better survival rate on SASP

McEntegart et al. 1996	200	SASP (100) Auranofin (100)	5 years	Randomized open study	31% on Rx at 5 years (15% on auranofin)	24% off SASP because of toxicity (cf 49 auranofin). Prompt resolution of side-effects on withdrawal	SASP more likely to be continued over 5 years with evidence of continuing benefit
Capell et al. 1998	200	SASP (102) PEN (98)	12 years	Randomized intention-to-treat	At 12 years DMARD use showed 32% of those alive and available for follow-up were on SASP 18% on D-penicillamine	Most toxicity occurred early, none was unexpected, all reversible	Sustained reduction in acute-phase response with sequential single DMARD
Summary comment						No drug-related deaths observed	

SASP do so because of a mucocutaneous reaction. Most episodes occur within the first six months, and may resolve with dose reduction.

Maculopapular   Most maculopapular reactions occur within the first two months of treatment; earlier occurrence may be due to prior sensitization. The pattern is similar to that of other drug exanthemata. Systemic symptoms are frequently absent. Drug withdrawal leads to resolution. Desensitization prior to starting SASP does not decrease the frequency of these reactions.

Fixed drug eruptions   These may occur, but are rare.

Urticaria   SASP urticaria is due to an allergic reaction rather than a direct pharmacological effect on mast cells. Rarely, concomitant angio-oedema can also occur.

Photosensitivity   In an RA patient on SASP with photosensitivity, drug-induced lupus needs to be considered. Nonsteroidal anti-inflammatory drugs (NSAIDs) are also known photosensitizers.

Major skin toxicity   Erythema multiforme, Stevens–Johnson syndrome and toxic epidermal necrolysis represent a continuum of mucocutaneous damage with similar histological features. In a review of all English language placebo-controlled and comparative published studies no cases were identified. However, anecdotal cases are recorded. In the inflammatory arthropathies, attributing these to SASP can be difficult as NSAIDs also cause such reactions. Rechallenge with SASP or a sulphonamide derivative such as a thiazide diuretic or a sulphylurea should be avoided.

Haematological

White blood cells   Reversible leucopenia due to SASP occurs in 1–3%, mostly in the first six months of therapy. Neutropenia is more common than lymphopenia.

Neutropenia   Neutropenia due to SASP can be fatal. In our experience, neutropenia improves without specific additional therapy, but episodes of life-threatening sepsis are reported. It is not known whether the neutropenia is due to immune-mediated damage to granulocyte precursors or peripheral neutrophil destruction. The response to granulocyte–monocyte colony-stimulating factor (GM-CSF) suggests that precursor damage occurs. Re-introduction of SASP or any sulphonamide is an absolute contraindication in those with a low previous neutrophil count attributed to SASP.

Lymphopenia   The mechanism of lymphopenia is not known. Drug withdrawal invariably results in normal levels. Our policy is to re-introduce SASP once levels are normal, with more frequent monitoring and dose adjustment to maintain a level above $0.7 \times 10^9/\text{L}$. Mild lymphopenia is accepted and monitored.

Red cells Megaloblastic anaemia due to SASP has been described but is rare, although an increase in the mean cell volume is reported in most series. In only a minority is this outside the normal range.

Macrocytosis is probably multifactorial. Despite the competitive antagonism between SASP and folic acid in the small bowel, folate levels in longitudinal studies remain within the normal range. In a minority there may be low-grade haemolysis. The SP component of SASP can cause oxidative damage to the red cell. This may occur to the cell membrane, haem may be oxidized to methaemoglobin and denatured globin may appear on the cell membrane as Heinz bodies. Such changes may result in haemolysis. Red cell glutathione protects the red cell from the damage of superoxide anions as oxygen is transferred from haemoglobin to tissues. Reduced glutathione levels are maintained by NADPH produced by aerobic glycolysis, therefore those with enzymatic defects in the hexose monophosphate shunt are more susceptible. Of these glucose-6-phosphate dehydrogenase (G6PD) is the most important to haemolysis. Caution in ethnic groups known to be at high risk of G6PD deficiency is advised.

Thrombocytopenia Three patients in a cohort of 1382 SASP-treated RA patients had a fall in platelet count. Of these one had a low platelet count prior to starting therapy; in the others it was difficult to be certain that SASP was the only responsible drug.

Bone marrow failure Cases of SASP and aplastic anaemia in RA have occurred. A causal association is difficult to prove, but the association between sulphonamides and aplastic anaemia is known. It is presumed to be an idiosyncratic reaction mediated by cytotoxic lymphocytes that secrete the inhibitory haemopoietic cytokines interferon-γ and tumour necrosis factor which impair haematopoiesis and stem cell apoptosis. No cases occurred in the cumulative literature outlined in Tables 1–4.

Neuropsychiatric Minor neuro-psychiatric reactions to SASP occur in 2% and may necessitate drug withdrawal. A causal association with the drug can be difficult to establish and premorbid factors may be contributory. Symptoms include irritability, anxiety headaches and an alteration in sleep pattern.

Hepatic Isolated minor rises in transaminases may occur in RA patients treated with SASP. Up to 3% of patients develop such abnormalities. Most reactions occur within the first 12 weeks of treatment and are not predictive of the rare more severe reactions. Withdrawal results in resolution, and drug rechallenge can lead to recurrence. These abnormalities are independent of dose and no disease or co-morbid factors have been identified to predict such abnormalities. Persistent or rising levels of transaminases may indicate either hepatic necrosis or a granulomatous hepatitis, both of which are reported with SASP.

Respiratory Respiratory reactions are rare. Most frequently described is an eosinophilic pneumonia, which occurs early in the course of treatment. Rash, fever, dyspnoea with pulmonary infiltrates and a peripheral eosinophilia are the typical presentation. In all reported cases resolution on drug withdrawal with appropriate supportive measures is documented. As this syndrome is also reported with sulphonamides the sulphapyridine component is implicated.

Immune-mediated reactions Although periorbital oedema, parotitis, ataxia, alopecia, peripheral neuropathy and hallucinations are reported with SASP in the British National Formulary, the authors and their colleagues have not observed these side-effects.

Hypogammaglobulinaemia

B-cell effects Reduced immunoglobulin levels occur in up to 10% of treated RA patients. IgM deficiency occurred in 5%, 3% had a selective fall in IgA levels and 2% a lone IgG level below the normal range. Continued SASP therapy resulted in resolution of a third of the IgM falls, but the low IgA and IgG levels remained. There were no infections, although the duration of follow-up was short.

Azoospermia

Azoospermia may occur during treatment but will reverse on withdrawal of therapy. Patients in a partnership where pregnancy is sought should be warned of this effect. The condition is not invariable—it cannot be relied on as a male contraceptive.

PRACTICAL PRESCRIBING

How to prescribe
- Provide patient and family doctor with written information about monitoring requirements, expected efficacy and strategies to minimize toxicity (see pp 50–51)
- Prescribe SASP EN tablets (the oval ones) to improve tolerability
- Increase dose slowly, usually by 0.5 g/week to minimize gastrointestinal tract toxicity
- Advise use of prochlorperazine if nausea is a problem in the first few weeks

cont.

- Warn patients of staining of soft contact lenses, alteration in colour of urine, sweat and tears (orange)
- Consider SASP suspension (250 mg/5 ml) if swallowing tablets is difficult
- Increase the dose if the initial effect wanes (to 40 mg/kg): average dose in prospective studies is 2.0–2.5 g daily
- Provide a monitoring card and ensure that patient (and carer) are aware of importance of sustained therapy and compliance with monitoring (most intensive in first six months)

■ TOXICITY MONITORING DURING SASP TREATMENT

As the vast majority of side-effects occur early during treatment, closer surveillance is advised in the first six months and less intensive assessment thereafter.

Guidelines for monitoring SASP Rx

At baseline
- Full blood count (FBC), urea and electrolytes (U&Es), liver function tests (LFTs), antinuclear antibodies (ANA)
- Education of patient, provision of monitoring card, written information to patient, shared care protocol to primary care provider

During initiation of therapy
- Fortnightly FBC for 12 weeks, then six-weekly to 24 weeks
- Six-weekly LFTs

Long term
- Three monthly FBC, U&Es, LFTs
- Patients should be advised to report unexplained fever, sore throat, bleeding, bruising or purpura
- ANA and double-stranded DNA should be repeated in cases of suspected drug-induced systemic lupus erythematosus (SLE)

PLANNING CONCEPTION

- Sulphasalazine can be used in women wishing to become pregnant but should be avoided in men wanting to father children in the near future

CONTRAINDICATIONS/CAUTIONS

- Known sulphonamide allergy
- Known G6PD deficiency
- Men wishing to father children in the near future (reversible fall in sperm count)

■ DRUG INTERACTIONS

Very few drug interactions have been reported with SASP. There is a possible interaction with cardiac glycosides—absorption of digoxin may be reduced. Enquiry about concomitant medication is therefore advisable.

SUMMARY

- SASP is a suitable first-choice DMARD in patients with active RA
- SASP improves markers of disease activity, physical function and quality of life, and reduces radiological progression of disease
- Serious toxicity is uncommon. Long-term studies have not shown any evidence of cumulative toxicity

SUMMARY STATEMENT

Patients selected for sulphasalazine should have:

- Active inflammatory disease either in terms of clinical evidence of inflammatory synovitis or laboratory evidence of an acute-phase response
- Seronegative and seropositive patients have been shown to respond and are equally suitable for selection

cont.

- All ages, men and women, may be expected to benefit, including children and the elderly
- All disease durations have been shown to respond, although sulphasalazine is commonly recommended as a disease-modifying drug early in the disease course

KEY REFERENCES

- McConkey 1980

- Pullar *et al*. 1983

- Capell *et al*. 1998

- Smolen *et al*. 1999

- Weinblatt 1999

■ SULPHASALAZINE—GP INFORMATION

Effect

Sulphasalazine is a disease-modifying antirheumatic drug (DMARD) used to treat rheumatoid arthritis, psoriatric arthritis and seronegative spondyloarthropathies. The onset of benefit is delayed 6–12 weeks. Two-thirds of patients will show significant improvement.

Prescribing

Target dose for your patient is _____mg.
- Use enteric coated tablets (sulphasalazine EN). These are better tolerated.
- Start 500 mg daily and increase the daily dose by 500 mg each week until a target dose of approximately 40 mg/kg is reached or side-effects occur.

Monitoring

- FBC, differential and urinalysis twice-weekly for the first three months.
- Then FBC, differential and urinalysis six-weekly until six months.
- Three-monthly thereafter.
- LFTs should be done monthly for the first three months and then six-monthly.
- Enter FBC, ESR and urinalysis on monitoring card.
- Check FBC if patient develops sore throat or abnormal bruising.

Contraindications

- Allergy to sulphonamides
- Men whose partners wish a pregnancy

Adverse effects and management

Nausea	Usually settles, prochloraperazine may be necessary initially
Rash	Stop treatment, usually does not recur on restarting
Mouth ulcers	Try Corlan pellets; if severe reduce dose
Fall in sperm count	Reversible on stopping drug. Potency not effected
Headache	Reduce dose if particularly troublesome
Haemolysis	Inform rheumatology unit if Hb <9 g/dL or MCV rising. Dose reduction may be necessary
Leucopenia, WCC <4	STOP therapy and contact rheumatology unit
Low platelets <150	STOP therapy and contact rheumatology unit
Hepatitis	Discuss raised ALT or AST with rheumatology unit. Accept moderate increase in αGT and alkaline phosphatase

Inform if Hb <9 g/dL

STOP SULPHASALAZINE AND CONTACT RHEUMATOLOGY UNIT IF:
- WCC <4 × 10^9/L
- Platelets <150 × 10^9/L
- AST and ALT are abnormal

Patient advice   The expected benefits and potential toxicity have been explained to your patient.

■ SULPHASALAZINE—PATIENT INFORMATION

It has been suggested that you start on sulphasalazine to help control your arthritis. Sulphasalazine is a disease-modifying antirheumatic drug which works by making arthritis less active and slows down damage to your joints. It may take 6–12 weeks before the sulphasalazine starts to work and you begin to feel better. You should not take sulphasalazine if you have had an allergic reaction to cotrimoxazole or septrin.

How do I take sulphasalazine?
■ The daily dose will be increased by one tablet every week until you reach your target dose of tablets. For the first week you will take one tablet daily, week 2 you will take 2 tablets daily, week 3 you will take 3 tablets daily and so on until you reach your target dose.
■ Sulphasalazine can be taken 2 or 3 times a day with or after food. The tablets should be swallowed whole and not crushed or chewed.
■ You should continue to take your other tablets as before.

What side-effects can these tablets cause?

Mild
■ Feeling sick tends to settle with time but an anti-sickness tablet may help. Diarrhoea, abdominal pain and frequent bowel movements may occur.
■ Urine may become more orange coloured and soft contact lenses may be stained.
■ Skin rash and mouth ulcers.

Rare
■ Blood problems—low white cell count (these fight infection), low platelets (these help to stop bruising/bleeding).
■ Abnormal tests of liver function.

These problems can be picked up early by regular blood checks.

If you should develop a sore throat, bruising, infection or fever, you should make an appointment to see your own doctor as soon as possible.

How often do I need to get my blood and urine checked?
■ Every 2 weeks for the first 3 months, 6-weekly for 6 months, and 3-monthly thereafter.
■ You will be given a monitoring card which you should bring with you to the clinic. Please ensure the results of all the tests are entered on the card.

Does sulphasalazine affect fertility or pregnancy?
■ Men whose partners wish to become pregnant should not take sulphasalazine because it can cause a fall in the sperm count. However, this gets better as soon as the drug is stopped. Pregnancy may still occur so contraception is still needed.
■ It is safer not to take sulphasalazine if you are pregnant or planning to become pregnant. Please discuss breast feeding with your doctor.

3 DMARDs

METHOTREXATE

> **KEY INDICATIONS**
> - Rheumatoid arthritis
> - Juvenile idiopathic arthritis
> - Psoriatic arthritis
> - Spondyloarthropathies

INTRODUCTION

Methotrexate (MTX) is used to treat a wide spectrum of rheumatological disorders, including rheumatoid arthritis (RA), psoriatic arthritis, Wegener's granulomatosis and systemic lupus erythematosus. However, RA remains the only arthropathy that is a licensed indication for treatment with MTX in the United Kingdom. The evidence base for the use of MTX in RA is stronger than for other rheumatological indications. In the treatment of RA, MTX has become established as the disease-modifying antirheumatic drug (DMARD) of first choice in many parts of the world (especially in North America and some parts of Europe). It has proved to be a cheap, effective and relatively well-tolerated drug. However, serious toxicity and fatalities have been reported, and MTX needs to be used with care, with appropriate arrangements for monitoring. Moreover, relatively few patients with RA have remission induced by MTX therapy and so, increasingly, MTX is used in combination with other conventional DMARDs or biologics (see Cytokine-Targeting Therapies on page 165).

PHARMACOLOGY

Methotrexate via its active metabolite 7-hydroxymethotrexate inhibits dihydrofolate reductase, preventing the reduction of dihydrofolate to tetrahydrofolate, which is a necessary step in the process of DNA synthesis. The inhibition of cell replication is a likely mode of action in the treatment of haematological malignancy, but whether this operates also in RA is not known. Numerous ex vivo activities have been reported using cells from RA patients, including the reduction of cytokine production, particularly interleukin (IL)-1 by peripheral blood mononuclear cell (PBMC) cultures, primarily from monocyte/macrophages, suppression of neutrophil activation, inhibition of neovascularization and hence angiogenesis. Matrix metalloproteinase (MMP) production may also be reduced relative to the tissue inhibitor of matrix metalloproteinase expression leading to net reduction in articular destruction. Novel enzyme targets have also been proposed, although these remain controversial. Inhibition of thymidylate synthetase has been reported. Stronger evidence for inhibition of 5-aminoimidazole-4-carboxamidoribonucleotide (AICAR) has been provided the net effect of which is to raise tissue expression of adenosine. Adenosine binds a variety of distinct adenosine receptors via which it mediates suppression of neutrophil adhesion, activation, leukotriene release, reduction in lymphocyte mitogen responses, reduced cytokine production by PBMC and reduced MMP release by synoviocytes.

■ BENEFIT

> ## EVIDENCE FOR BENEFIT IN RA
>
> Table 1 shows evidence for benefit of MTX compared with placebo
> Table 2 shows comparative studies with other DMARDs
> Table 3 shows selected studies in which radiographic outcomes have been measured

MTX monotherapy

The efficacy of MTX in the treatment of RA was first established in four placebo-controlled randomized trials. These studies clearly established that MTX was superior to placebo in the short-term treatment of RA (see Table 1). Subsequent studies in the past decade have compared MTX with several other commonly used DMARDs (see Table 2) in which key studies are summarized. The Leflunomide RA Investigators Group trial that compared placebo, leflunomide and MTX provides typical results; the improvements in disease activity, physical function, quality of life and radiological progression are shown in Figure 1. Approximately 50% of patients might be expected to have some clinical benefit around the ACR 20% response level.

Numerous double-blind randomized controlled trials have compared MTX with other DMARDs (vs sulphasalazine—SASP, SASP/MTX, azathioprine, auranofin, gold, leflunomide and etanercept). Prospective double-blind randomized controlled trials confirmed that MTX has comparable efficacy to SASP, etanercept (in early RA), leflunomide and intramuscular (IM) gold (in established disease). MTX is superior in efficacy to azathioprine and auranofin. No direct comparisons have been made with hydroxychloroquine, penicillamine, cyclosporin or infliximab. These findings are in keeping with the results of a meta-analysis that concluded that IM gold, penicillamine, SASP and MTX have

Table 1 Early randomized controlled trials/meta-analysis comparing methotrexate with placebo in rheumatoid arthritis

Reference	Comparator drug	Disease	Study design	Follow-up	Outcome efficacy	Outcome toxicity	Comment
Weinblatt et al. 1985	Placebo	RA	Double-blind, randomized cross-over (n = 28)	24 week	Superior to placebo	LFTs, nausea, diarrhoea	Short-term efficacy proven
Andersen et al. 1985	Placebo	RA	Double-blind, randomized cross-over (n = 12)	13 weeks	Superior to placebo	—	Immunological analysis revealed no significant changes
Thompson et al. 1984	Placebo	RA	Randomized, controlled, parenteral (n = 48)	6 weeks	Superior to placebo	—	
Williams et al. 1985	Placebo	RA	Randomized multi-centre, controlled (n = 189)	18 weeks	Superior to placebo	As above	
Tugwell 1987	Placebo	RA	Meta-analysis of above studies	—	Superior to placebo	As above	Confirmed efficacy in DMARD-resistant RA

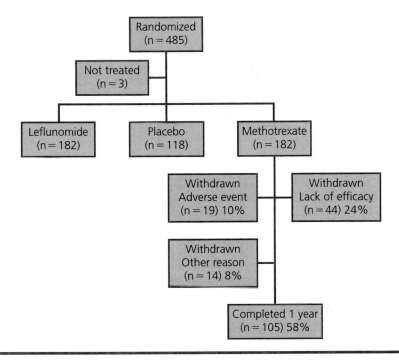

Figure 1 Treatment of active rheumatoid arthritis with leflunomide compared with placebo and methotrexate. The Leflunomide Rheumatoid Arthritis Investigators Group. *Arch Intern Med 1999; 159:2542–2550.*

similar efficacy. The requirement for folic acid or folinic acid was also addressed with respect to effects on efficacy and reduction of toxicity (see Table 2). Data suggest that supplementation is effective in reducing toxicity and has no meaningful effect on efficacy, although slightly higher doses of MTX may be required.

Radiology

MTX is effective in reducing the rate of articular damage in RA as assessed by radiographic progression. Several comparisons with other DMARDs suggest that MTX is at least as effective as SASP, leflunomide and gold in reducing progression.

Table 2 Key comparative randomized controlled trials using methotrexate in rheumatoid arthritis

Reference	Comparator drug	Disease	Study design	Follow-up	Outcome efficacy	Outcome toxicity	Comment
Haagsma et al. 1997	MTX vs SASP vs MTX/SASP	Early RA	Double-blind RCT	1 year	Equal efficacy	Nausea more common with combination	SASP and MTX have equivalent efficacy/toxicity in early RA
Dougados et al. 1999	MTX vs SASP vs MTX/SASP	Early RA	Double-blind RCT	1 year	Equal efficacy	Nausea more common with combination	SASP and MTX have equivalent efficacy/toxicity in early RA
Shiroky et al. 1993	MTX vs MTX/folinic acid	RA	Double-blind RCT	1 year	Equal efficacy	Toxicity reduced with folinic acid	Use of folinic acid reduces MTX toxicity without reducing efficacy
Morgan et al. 1990	MTX vs MTX/folic acid	RA	Double-blind RCT	6 months	Equal efficacy	Toxicity reduced with folic acid	Use of folic acid reduces MTX toxicity without reducing efficacy
van Ede et al. 2001	MTX vs MTX/folinic acid vs MTX/folic acid	RA	Double-blind RCT	12 months	Higher dose for equivalent efficacy in folinic acid / folate recipients	Primarily hepatic toxicity reduced by folic acid or folinic acid	Use of folic acid (daily) or folinic acid (weekly) reduces MTX toxicity
Jeurissen et al. 1991	MTX vs AZA	RA	Double-blind RCT	1 year	MTX superior to AZA	MTX better tolerated than AZA	MTX is more effective than azathioprine, and better tolerated

Weinblatt et al. 1993	MTX vs auranofin	RA	Double-blind RCT	9 months	MTX superior to Aur for radiographic outcome		Methotrexate is more effective than auranofin
Rau et al. 1991	MTX vs IM gold	RA	Double-blind RCT	6 months	Equal efficacy		MTX and IM gold have equal efficacy, but MTX is better tolerated
Strand et al. 1999	MTX vs LEF vs placebo	RA	Double-blind RCT	1 year	Equal efficacy		MTX and LEF have equivalent efficacy and toxicity
Bathon et al. 2000	MTX vs etanercept	Early RA	Double-blind RCT	1 year	Equal efficacy Little radiographic progression on MTX	Fewer adverse events with etanercept	In early RA, MTX is as effective as etanercept

Two-year data suggest marginal benefit for etanercept over MTX upon direct comparison. Selected studies are summarized in Table 3.

Long-term studies

More patients continue MTX therapy in the long term than other DMARDs, with fewer patients stopping treatment because of inefficacy and toxicity. Maetzel *et al.* (2000) found that 36% of patients continued on MTX therapy for more than five years, compared to 22% treated with SASP, and 23% treated with IM gold. Others have reported higher levels of MTX retention up to 60% over five years in prospective studies.

■ HARM

Toxicity in RA

Approximately 20% of patients receiving MTX will develop a side-effect. The commonest adverse events are shown in Table 4. Nausea and oral ulceration may be significant but usually respond to local or symptomatic therapy. Serious and life-threatening toxicity is uncommon, but several deaths have been reported in prospective clinical trials or in case reports. Opportunistic infection occurs rarely, but can be fatal. The following areas merit particular emphasis.

Hepatic toxicity   Transaminase elevation is variable in practice but occurs in approximately 10% of MTX-treated patients in clinical trials. Clinically significant hepatic disease is rare (1/1000 per five years' treatment). Folic acid or folinic acid supplementation reduces hepatic toxicity. Risk factors for liver damage include age, treatment duration and total MTX dose and diabetes mellitus. Persistent elevation of transaminases despite dose reduction or discontinuation of MTX indicates further investigation. This may include liver biopsy even if ultrasound (US), magnetic resonance imaging (MRI) or computed tomography (CT) scans are normal.

Pulmonary   Pulmonary symptoms may occur at any time during therapy but are more common early; 50% of episodes occur within eight months of starting therapy. Many cases have subacute onset over weeks rather than days. A high degree of suspicion should therefore be maintained. No risk factors are conclusively recognized, although some reports suggest that age, diabetes mellitus, hypoalbuminaemia, substantial previous DMARD use and RA pulmonary disease may be predisposing factors. Symptoms include nonproductive cough, fever, fatigue and dyspnoea, and may be difficult to distinguish from infection. Early management should therefore cover both diagnostic possibilities. High-resolution CT scan and, if necessary, biopsy may be necessary to confirm the diagnosis. Immunosuppression and ventilatory support may be necessary pending individual progress. Rechallenge with MTX is not recommended.

Table 3 Radiographic progression on methotrexate in rheumatoid arthritis

Reference	Comparator drugs	Disease	Study design	Follow-up	Outcome	Comment
Genovese et al. 2002	MTX vs etanercept	Early RA	RCT, double-blind. Sharp scale	2 years	Etanercept better than MTX in reducing progression	
Rau et al. 2002	MTX vs GST	RA	Open extension of RCT	3 years	MTX and GST reduced the slope of radiographic progression	MTX and GST similar in effect on erosion
Cohen et al. 2001	MTX vs LEF vs placebo	RA	RCT, double-blind: patients continuing into year 2	2 year	Sustained reduction in radiographic progression	MTX and LEF similar effect on radiographic progression
Sharp et al. 2000	MTX vs SASP vs LEF vs placebo	RA	Combined analysis of 3 RCT	1 year	MTX, LEF, SASP all better than placebo	MTX, SASP and LEF similar in effect
Strand et al. 1999	MTX vs LEF vs placebo	RA	RCT, double-blind. Sharp score	1 year	MTX and LEF better than placebo in reducing radiographic progression	MTX and LEF probably similar in effect on radiographic progression
Dougados et al. 1999	MTX vs SASP vs MTX / SASP	Early RA	RCT, double-blind. Modified Sharp score	1 year	Modest progression in Sharp score; all groups similar	No placebo comparison
Weinblatt et al. 1993	MTX vs auranofin	RA	Double-blind RCT	9 months	Reduced radiological progression with MTX	MTX is more effective than auranofin
Jeurissen et al. 1991	MTX vs AZA	RA	RCT, double-blind. Sharp scale	1 year	Less radiographic progression in MTX group	MTX is superior to AZA in reducing erosion

Table 4 Toxicity of methotrexate in rheumatoid arthritis

Adverse event	Frequency	Timescale and nature	Clinical management
Infections	Common	Any time; opportunistic infections reported, but rare	Continue treatment during minor infection; suspend therapy in severe or opportunistic infection
Gastrointestinal Nausea/vomiting Oral ulcers Anorexia Dyspepsia	Common	Dose related	Oral antiemetics may be effective; try dose reduction; conversion to parenteral administration often effective
Alopecia	Uncommon	Idiosyncratic	Dose reduction; cessation of therapy if severe
Haematological Leucopenia Neutropenia Reduced platelets Anaemia	Uncommon	Idiosyncratic, sometimes dose related. Increased risk in elderly, renal impairment or with co-prescription of another antifolate drug. Leucopenia is commoner than suppression of other cell lines	Suspend therapy if there is any sudden drop in WCC or platelets, if neutrophils <2 × 10^9/L, total WCC <4 × 10^9/L, or platelets <150 × 10^9/L. If neutrophils <0.5 × 10^9/L provide full supportive therapy, and "rescue" with IV folinic acid
Pneumonitis	Uncommon	Idiosyncratic; usually within first year of treatment. Patients should report any unexplained dyspnoea or cough. May have peripheral blood eosinophilia	Withdraw therapy; oral prednisolone 60 mg daily may hasten recovery
Rash	Rare	Idiosyncratic	Dose reduction; cessation of therapy if severe
Hepatic fibrosis	Very rare	Cumulative; risk may be increased in obesity, elderly, alcohol ingestion	Withdraw therapy if AST/ALT increase to > x3 ULN; reduce dose and/or monitor closely for minor elevations of AST/ALT; withdraw therapy or perform liver biopsy if even mild elevations are persistent

Common   1–10% of patients
Uncommon   0.1–1%
Rare   0.01–0.1%
Very rare 0.01%

Haematological Leucopenia, thrombocytopenia and anaemia are all reported with MTX but are not common. Increased risk arises in renal failure or pre-existing folate deficiency. Most episodes respond to drug cessation, although severe marrow suppression may require supportive management including use of colony stimulating factors and erythropoietin. Severe leucopenia (e.g. neutrophil count $< 0.05 \times 10^9$) may respond to folinic acid "rescue". Severe marrow suppression is associated with fatality.

Malignancies MTX may act as a co-inducer of malignancy. Most studies suggest, however, that the risk of malignancy in MTX-treated patients is not elevated above that of patients with RA who already carry a marginally increased risk. Several case reports suggest that B-cell lymphomas, often associated with Epstein–Barr virus, may occur more commonly and characteristically regress on discontinuation of MTX.

Nodulosis Increased numbers of nodules occurring at both common and atypical sites are reported in MTX recipients. Ulceration and infection may complicate these lesions.

■ PRACTICAL PRESCRIBING

Practical advice on prescribing MTX is shown in Table 5.

Monitoring during MTX treatment

Patients should be given oral and written information about MTX therapy, and the potential for side-effects. Patients should be advised to seek medical help in the event of unexplained fever, sore throat, bleeding, bruising, rash, jaundice, cough or breathlessness. The British Society of Rheumatology (BSR) has produced guidelines for the monitoring of MTX therapy in the treatment of RA (see Table 6). Results should be entered on a monitoring card that remains with the patient.

Drug interactions

Important drug interactions are shown in Table 7.

Vaccination policy

Live vaccines should not be administered.

Table 5 Practical guide to prescribing methotrexate in rheumatoid arthritis

Dose		
Initial dose:	5–7.5 mg/week	Reduce dose in elderly and in renal impairment. The effective dose varies, and occasionally >25 mg/week may be required. Benefit is seen after 8–12 weeks of therapy. Splitting the dose into 3 equal doses taken at 12-hour intervals may reduce side-effects in some patients
Increments:	2.5–5 mg/week each month	
Target dose:	15–25 mg/week	
Be aware that 2.5 mg and 10 mg tablets appear similar—advise patients to check tablet strength		
Folic acid	5 mg/week	Dose and timing are probably not critical
Parenteral use	Subcutaneous or intramuscular administration can be used	The bioavailability of oral methotrexate varies between patients. Parenteral administration can be tried in patients with a suboptimal response to oral methotrexate, or to minimize GI side-effects
Contraindications	Folate deficiency Methotrexate hypersensitivity Severe renal impairment Hepatic disease Bone marrow suppression Alcohol addiction	
Cautions	Elderly Pleural effusions, ascites Pulmonary disease Mild renal impairment	Toxicity is increased in the elderly. Methotrexate enters pleura/ascitic fluid slowly, and leaves it slowly, with potential for increased toxicity. Detection of pneumonitis is more difficult in patients with pre-existing pulmonary disease
Alcohol	Advise moderation	Abstention is probably not required, but patients should be advised to be very moderate in their alcohol intake
Pregnancy	Contraindicated	Methotrexate is teratogenic. Conception must be avoided during therapy and for three months after stopping therapy in female patients and partners of male patients
Breast feeding	Contraindicated	

Table 6   BSR guidelines for monitoring methotrexate

Chest X-ray	Baseline	Repeat if the patient reports unexplained cough or dyspnoea
Full blood count	Baseline Weekly until dose is stable Monthly thereafter	Check B_{12} and folate if macrocytosis noted
AST/ALT	Baseline Weekly until dose is stable Monthly thereafter	Avoid methotrexate in patients with pre-existent liver disease. Check hepatitis viral serology in patients at high risk
Urea and creatinine	Baseline Every 6–12 months	Methotrexate is 90% excreted via the kidneys. If there is mild renal impairment, reduce dose. Avoid methotrexate in moderate/severe renal impairment

Table 7   Important drug interactions with methotrexate

Antifolate drugs	Phenytoin, trimethoprim, co-trimoxazole, triamterene, Fansidar, Maloprim	Avoid all other antifolate drugs, although sulphasalazine has been widely used in combination with methotrexate and appears to be safe
Competition for renal excretion	NSAIDs, sulphonamides, penicillins, probenecid	
Drugs that impair renal function	NSAIDs, ACE inhibitors, cyclosporin	Although many RA patients do continue on NSAID and take an ACE inhibitor, combination studies with cyclosporin are reported
Drugs that displace MTX from protein binding	NSAIDs, sulphonamides, hypoglycaemics, tetracyclines, chloramphenicol, etretinates	Methotrexate is >50% protein bound

SUMMARY

- Methotrexate is a suitable "first choice" DMARD in patients with active RA.
- Methotrexate improves disease activity, physical function and quality of life, and reduces radiological progression.
- Serious toxicity is uncommon, but careful monitoring is required to minimize risk.

KEY REFERENCES

- Strand *et al.* 1999

- Haagsma *et al.* 1997

- Felson 1992

- Maetzel *et al.* 2000

- Sharp *et al.* 2000

METHOTREXATE—GP INFORMATION SHEET

Methotrexate is used to treat RA, psoriatic arthritis and some connective tissue diseases. Toxicity can occur but, if certain precautions are taken, most patients tolerate methotrexate without serious problems. It may take 8–12 weeks before an effect is seen.

Prescribing
- The usual starting dose is 5–7.5 mg per *week* taken every Sunday.
- The usual increase in weekly dose is 2.5–5 mg every 4 weeks, until a response is seen, or side-effects occur. Usual maximum dose is 25 mg/week.
- Splitting the dose so that it is taken at 8–12 hourly intervals may reduce the incidence of side-effects in some patients.

Be aware of similar appearance of 2.5 mg and 10 mg tablets. Ask patient to check tablet strength dispensed.

Patients will still need their NSAID and analgesic drugs, although these can sometimes be stopped/reduced if/when the patient responds to methotrexate.

Folic acid supplements: Please prescribe folic acid 5 mg/week, to be taken mid-week.

Alcohol: Moderation (e.g. <7 units alcohol/week) or abstention from alcohol is advised.

Absolute contraindications: Hepatic disease, pregnancy or planned pregnancy, moderate/severe renal impairment.

Cautions: Mild renal impairment, respiratory disease and co-prescription of drugs that may may interfere with renal function (NSAIDs, diuretics, ACE inhibitors, etc.). Alcohol ingestion.

Drug interactions: Folate antagonists (co-trimoxazole, trimethoprim, triamterene, phenytoin, Fansidar, Maloprim) must not be co-prescribed. Some other drugs reduce methotrexate excretion or displace it from its protein binding—check the BNF.

Blood monitoring
We would be grateful for your help in monitoring this therapy.
We suggest:
- Baseline CXR (will be arranged in hospital)
- FBC/diff—weekly until dose is stable, thereafter every 4 weeks
- LFT—weekly until dose is stable, thereafter every 4 weeks
- U&E—every 3–6 months

Toxicity: Bone marrow suppression may occur, and this may be precipitated by renal impairment or co-prescription of another folate antagonist. During any illness associated with infection or potential dehydration, methotrexate should be withheld and FBC and U&E checked.

Side-effects	Action
Nausea/vomiting	Try splitting the dose into three parts at 12-hour intervals; antiemetics; may need dose reduction; consider parenteral methotrexate
Oral ulcers	Try Corlan pellets; reduce dose if necessary
White cell counts $<4 \times 10^9$/L, PMN $<2 \times 10^9$/L	Stop methotrexate and contact rheumatology unit
Platelet count $<150 \times 10^9$/L	Stop methotrexate and contact rheumatology unit
Haemoglobin <9 g/dL	Check haematinics and contact rheumatology unit
AST/ALT are high	Stop methotrexate and restart after LFTs return to normal
AST/ALT >3 times ULN	Stop methotrexate and contact rheumatology unit
Renal function deteriorates	Discuss with rheumatology unit—may need dose reduction
Unexplained cough/dyspnoea	Stop methotrexate and arrange CXR

Patient advice The patients have been given an information sheet about the expected benefits and potential side-effects of methotrexate therapy.

3 DMARDs

Sodium aurothiomalate

> **KEY INDICATIONS**
> - Rheumatoid arthritis
> - Psoriatic arthritis (less common)

■ INTRODUCTION

Gold compounds have a long pedigree in the treatment of rheumatoid arthritis (RA) dating back to 1929 when Forestier used gold salts on the basis that they had an antituberculous effect and therefore might be useful in chronic arthritis (Forestier 1929). Gold was the mainstay in the treatment of RA until the advent of sulphasalazine, methotrexate and other newer DMARDs. The two most commonly used gold compounds are an injectable form as disodium aurothiomalate (Myocrisin®) and an orally administered compound triethylphosphine gold (auranofin). Both drugs have a DMARD effect but are not equipotent.

■ PHARMACOLOGY

Aurothiomalate is water soluble and is rapidly absorbed after intramuscular injection with peak levels after three hours. Gold is highly protein bound and is primarily concentrated in the recticuloendothelial system with the highest concentrations being found in the liver, bone marrow, lymph nodes, skin and muscle. Relatively smaller amounts are found in synovial tissue unless there is active inflammation, when gold is localized within synovial membrane macrophages in inclusion bodies known as "aurosomes". Gold excretion is via the urine and faeces, but gold can be detected in the body for up to 25 years after treatment has ceased.

■ MODE OF ACTION

The precise mode of action of gold compounds in inflammatory joint disease is not known, but an interaction with thiol (-SH) groups on proteins and cell membranes is thought to be important (Jeon et al. 2000). In-vitro and in-vivo effects on macrophage function, B-cell function and signal transduction have all been observed.

Effects

- Inhibition of NFκβ activation
- Inhibition of B-cell activation
- Inhibition of osteoclastic bone resorption
- IL-1ra production increased

■ BENEFIT

Sodium aurothiomalate (GST) has a DMARD effect and has been shown to be equipotent with sulphasalazine, methotrexate and D-penicillamine (Felson *et al.* 1990) in meta-analyses. It is more effective than auranofin (see p. 80). Long-term retention of gold is not as good as methotrexate, because of increased patient withdrawal because of side-effects.

EVIDENCE OF BENEFIT IN RA

Table 1 shows the evidence for clinical benefit against placebo
Table 2 shows clinical comparison with other DMARDs
Table 3 shows evidence from radiological studies
Table 4 shows long-term studies

Injectable gold has been studied over many years: indeed Fraser conducted a study in 1945 in Glasgow that demonstrated clinical benefit. In 1960, the Empire Rheumatism Council concluded a placebo-controlled study in 199 patients over 12–18 months and demonstrated clinical and laboratory benefit with relatively low toxicity (only 14% stopped IM gold because of adverse events). In part this low figure may reflect the dearth of alternative drugs at that time.

Subsequent placebo-controlled and comparative studies of GST shown in Tables 1 and 2 have demonstrated the impressive efficacy of GST, but almost all have found toxicity withdrawals of 30–40%.

Typical findings are those of Rau *et al.* (1997) who, in a 12-month study comparing IM gold with methotrexate, reported on outcome in 174 patients with active early erosive RA; 24% of the gold-treated group and 11% of the methotrexate group achieved remission. An improvement of >50% in swollen and tender joints and erythrocyte sedimentation rate (ESR) was seen in 76% of gold- and 68% of methotrexate-treated patients. Significantly more patients were withdrawn from the gold cohort because of toxicity (37% compared with 7% in those on methotrexate). Therefore, while more patients achieved remission with gold, tolerability was better with methotrexate.

Similar results were found in a Glasgow study where over 48 weeks 43% of gold- and 19% of methotrexate-treated patients were withdrawn because of toxicity.

Effect on radiological progression

IM gold has been shown to have an effect on delaying the progression of radiological erosions.

In the Rau study over 36 months, both gold and methotrexate reduced the slope of radiographic progression in parallel with clinical improvement. No difference between gold and methotrexate was shown at 12 and 18 months but some advantage was shown for parenteral gold at 36 months (Rau et al. 1998).

These effects were further demonstrated in other studies (Rau et al. 2002) and assessed in a review of three studies (van Riel et al. 1995a) and a review of gold compounds on radiographic progression in RA (Sanders 2000).

■ LONG-TERM STUDIES (Table 4)

In a study of 541 RA patients 119 received IM gold and 34% remained on gold at 5 years (Jessop et al. 1998). No deaths were attributed to gold. Adverse reactions led to treatment withdrawal in 48 patients (40 mucocutaneous, five proteinuria, two thrombocytopenia, one diarrhoea).

Munro et al. (1998) studied 440 RA patients and found that 36% remained on treatment at five years. Those treated early (< 2 years' disease duration) had better functional outcomes as measured by the Health Assessment Questionnaire at 5 years. Significant improvement in all other parameters of disease activity regardless of disease duration was seen at five years.

A Finnish study (Lehtinen et al. 1991) of 573 patients treated at hospital for the first time between 1961 and 1966 showed that gold therapy was not associated with premature death—indeed gold treatment was associated with a high survival rate.

A Swedish study over 10 years (retrospective) in 376 patients showed 26% on treatment at five years but only 8% at year 10 (Bendix et al. 1996).

Side-effects, especially mucocutaneous, were the most common reasons for cessation of therapy over the first four years, and inefficacy the most prominent reason in the later years of assessment. No patients were noted to have died. All side-effects reversed.

Compliance issues

An advantage of injectable gold is that drug administration is assured and the patient is simultaneously able to co-operate with monitoring.

■ HARM

Gold compounds result in more toxicity than most DMARDs; Table 5 lists the most common side-effects. Withdrawal rate because of toxicity is approximately 30% in the first year.

Table 1 Placebo controlled studies of intramuscular gold in RA

Reference	n	Comparative drugs	Study design/disease duration	Duration of follow-up (months)	Outcome efficacy	Outcome toxicity	Conclusion/comment
Empire Rheumatism Council 1960	199	GST/placebo	Randomized double-blind controlled (disease duration – 1/3 <3 years: 2/3 3–5 years)	12–18	Significant clinical and laboratory benefit with GST cf placebo	14% stopped GST due to toxicity 4 cases severe dermatitis	GST effective in the treatment of RA Incidence of toxicity low in this study
Cooperating Clinics Committee of ARC 1973	68	GST/placebo	Randomized double-blind controlled (extension randomized crossover of GST-treated patients) (disease duration – 1/3 each of <3 years: 3–5 years: >5 years)	6 (24)	Significant improvement in ESR and physician global with GST. Trend towards improvement in number of synovitic joints with GST	33% stopped GST due to toxicity	GST may suppress synovitis. Toxicity common. Numbers in 24-month follow-up too small for analysis
Sigker et al. 1974	27	GST/placebo	Randomized double-blind controlled. (median disease duration 3 years)	24	Significant improvement in clinical parameters with GST cf placebo. Slowing of radiographic progression with GST	No data given	GST effective DMARD. No ESR data. Unable to comment on safety

Pullar et al. 1983	90	GST/SASP/placebo	Randomized, GST open, SASP/placebo blinded. (6-9 year disease duration)	6	Significant clinical and laboratory benefit from GST and SASP. Placebo: no benefit	37% stopped GST due to toxicity All side-effects reversed	GST effective DMARD but toxicity common
Ward et al. 1983	193	GST/auranofin/ placebo	Randomized double-blind controlled. ITT (mean disease duration 5 years)	5	GST and auranofin # superior to placebo. 35% GST group had clinically important improvement in pain/ tenderness	29% stopped GST due to toxicity 1 pneumonitis - responded to steroid	GST and auranofin equally effective treatments for RA. More toxicity with GST
Capell et al. 1986	90	GST/auranofin/ placebo	Randomized	36	More rapid benefit with GST. Inefficacy withdrawals 3% GST 47% auranofin 90% placebo	30% GST 17% auranofin Toxicity withdrawals All reversed	Sustained GST response over 36 months
Williams et al. 1988	186	GST/SASP/placebo	Double-blind randomized	37	GST similar to SASP	SASP better tolerated 41% off GST 16% off SASP because of side-effects	Placebo response greater than in other similar studies

Table 2 Intramuscular gold in RA: Comparative studies (randomized monotherapy)

Reference	n	Comparative drugs	Study design/ disease duration	Duration of follow-up (months)	Outcome efficacy	Outcome toxicity	Conclusion/comment
Suarez-Almazor et al. 1988	40	GST/IM MTX	Randomized double-blind (disease duration: ~ 50% <2 years: ~50% 2–10 years)	6	Significant improvement in all clinical and laboratory parameters with GST. Similar efficacy to MTX	Significantly more toxicity with GST. Toxicity withdrawals 35%	GST effective but more toxicity in short term cf MTX
Morassut et al. 1989	35	GST/oral MTX	Randomized double-blind (mean disease duration 5.7 years)	6	Significant improvement in all variables with GST. Trend towards earlier response with MTX GST ≡ MTX	35% stopped GST due to toxicity. All side-effects reversed	Both GST and MTX effective in short-term treatment of RA
Rau et al. 1997	174	GST/IM MTX	Randomized double-blind. ITT (disease duration: 83% <3years: 61% <1 year)	12	GST and IM MTX both effective. Significantly more remissions with GST (24%) cf MTX (11%)	37% stopped GST due to toxicity. 25% of toxicity withdrawals achieved remission	Higher rate of remission than other studies. Dose of GST higher than other studies

Zeidler et al. 1998	375	GST/cyclosporin A	Randomized open. ITT Blinded radiological endpoint (mean disease duration 1 year)	18	Significant improvement in all clinical variables. GST ≡ cyclosporin A. No difference in radiological outcome between groups	35% stopped GST due to toxicity. Most withdrawals in first 6 months	GST effective in early disease. Toxicity common
Menninger et al. 1998	174	GST/IM MTX	2 year open extension of Rau et al. 1997	36	GST and IM MTX equivalent efficacy. 61% GST treated ≥ moderate response per DAS (ITT analysis)	52% stopped GST due to toxicity	High rate of remission maintained over 3 years
Hamilton et al. 2001	141	GST/oral MTX	Randomized open. ITT (2–15 year disease duration: median 6 years)	12	GST effective, equivalent to oral MTX. 18% GST patients achieved inactivation of disease	43% stopped GST due to toxicity	Response rates for GST and MTX low compared with other studies. MTX dose low

Table 3 Radiology studies of intramuscular gold

Reference	No. studies reviewed	Comparator drugs	Conclusion
van Riel et al. 1995	3	SASP, MTX, Auranofin, HCQ, azathioprine	IM gold, SASP, MTX slow radiographic progression, others do not
Sanders 2000	8	Antimalarials	IM gold better than placebo in slowing erosions. Antimalarials not effective
Rau et al. 2002	1	MTX	Both gold and MTX reduce slope of radiographic progression over 3 years of follow-up

Mucocutaneous

Gold rashes may be dramatic, especially those that occur early in treatment. Recurrence is not invariable. A lower dose or longer intervals between injections may be worth trying. Late rashes are often more localized and scaling. These tend not to settle (and not to deteriorate greatly). Many patients who are deriving a good effect from IM gold are willing to tolerate such rashes. The same is true of mild mouth ulceration. More severe ulceration interfering with eating and speech usually necessitates drug withdrawal.

Fortunately, exfoliative dermatitis is extremely rare. However, affected patients are often acutely unwell and require admission for supportive therapy which may include IV fluids and hydrocortisone. Rechallenge is contraindicated.

Nitritoid reactions

Episodes of flushing (similar to that noted with nitrates, hence the name) tend to occur after the first few injections and then diminish and settle entirely. These reactions are possibly more common when ACE inhibitions are co-prescribed.

There is no evidence that they predict more serious toxicity, and most patients are willing to continue therapy when explanation for symptoms is given.

Proteinuria

If urine dipstix reveals more than a trace of protein, the following procedure is suggested:

■ Repeat: if still positive →
■ MSSU (mid-stream specimen of urine): if negative →
■ 24 hour quantitative protein: if >0.5 g/L stop gold
■ Abdominal ultrasound and renal biopsy may be necessary

Table 4 Long term studies of intramuscular gold in RA

Reference	n	Comparative drugs	Study design/ disease duration	Duration of follow-up	Outcome efficacy	Outcome toxicity	Conclusion/comment
Lehtinen et al. 1991	573	"No gold" group	Retrospective	23–28 years	Compared with patients not treated with gold high survival rate on IM gold	Most side-effects early	Gold treatment not associated with premature death
Bendix et al. 1996	376	None	Retrospective cohort	10 years	Inefficacy late cause of discontinuation	No serious side-effects. Mucocutaneous early	26% on Rx at 5 years, 8% at 10 years
Jessop et al. 1998	541	GST/penicillamine/ HCQ/auranofin	Randomized open (median disease duration 2 years)	60 years	34% remaining on GST at 5 years. Equivalent to HCQ and auranofin. Significantly less cf penicillamine	41% stopped GST due to toxicity	GST has sustained efficacy in RA. Toxicity commonest reason for stopping treatment
Munro et al. 1998	440	None	Continuation of prospective study	5 years	Significant improvement in pain, Ritchie Index, ESR, CRP. Function only improved at 5 years in those treated early	62% withdrew from study because of toxicity (reversible). No deaths due to GST	Treating patients early maximizes functional response at 5 years

- Gold-induced dermatitis is common and is dose related. A rising eosinophil count may herald an exfoliative dermatitis, but this is rare, and more often than not the raised eosinophil count is a feature of increased disease activity in the early phases of treatment. Patients should be carefully questioned about skin rash as they often conceal this if they are responding well to the gold.
- A nitritoid reaction occurs early in treatment and is associated with hypotension, sweating and occasional fainting. Ideally, patients should wait in the consulting room for 30 minutes after their gold injection prior to going home. Reassure patient and GP that the effect will diminish with continued therapy.

Pregnancy

Information on the effects of aurothiomalate on human pregnancy is insufficient and it therefore is prudent to discontinue gold therapy when pregnancy is recognized (Ostensen 2001). In patients on gold trying to fall pregnant, a four-weekly injection schedule can allow patients to have treatment when menstruation begins, and gold is withheld if the menstrual period is delayed.

SUMMARY

- Intramuscular gold therapy is an effective DMARD in the therapy of RA.
- Long-term continuation is a problem because of side-effects such as skin rash.
- Careful monitoring is required even in patients on long-term therapy.

KEY REFERENCES

- Fraser 1945

- Bendix *et al.* 1996

- Capell *et al.* 1986

- Munro *et al.* 1998

- Lehtinen *et al.* 1991

■ INTRAMUSCULAR GOLD (MYOCRISIN) INJECTIONS—GP INFORMATION

Injectable gold therapy is of proven benefit as a second-line agent in rheumatoid arthritis and psoriatic arthritis. Onset of action is 2–6 months.

Prescribing
- Gold should be administered as a deep intramuscular injection to the buttock or upper thigh.
- Start with a 10 mg test dose (this will often be given in the clinic).
- The follwing week give 50 mg and continue 50 mg injections weekly for 20 weeks or until the patient responds (usually 2–6 months) or develops side-effects.
- The frequency of injections will be reduced if/when the patient responds.

If there is no response at 6 months or if a loss of effect occurs, then 100 mg weekly for 6–10 weeks may be suggested by the clinic. NSAIDs and analgestics should be continued, although these may be reduced or stopped once the patient responds to treatment.

Monitoring
- Enquire about skin rash/mouth ulcers before each injection.
- Check FBC, differential, white cell count and urinalysis before each injection and enter the results (including ESR) on the monitoring card. However, if this is not possible, blood may be taken at the same time as gold is given, *so long as* the result is checked *prior* to the next administration of gold.

Toxicity
Stop treatment and contact clinic if:
- WCC $<4\times10^9$/L
- Platelets $<150\times10^9$/L
- Urine protein + or more (see below)
- Severe rash or mouth ulceration

Adverse effects	Management
Rash	If mild may respond to dose reduction, otherwise stop gold. Exfoliative dermatitis may rarely develop
Pruritus, no rash	Try antihistamine, reduce dose
Mouth ulcers	Try Corlan® pellets, decrease dose or stop if severe
Vasomotor (flushing, hypotension)	?more frequent in patients on ACE inhibitors. Reduce dose and give injection in recumbent position
Leucopenia ($<4\times10^9$/L)	STOP treatment and contact clinic
Low platelets <150	STOP treatment and contact clinic
Proteinuria (+)	Withhold injections, check MSSU. Clinic will arrange 24-hour collection if negative

Patient advice   *The expected benefits and potential toxicity have been explained to your patient.*

Contraindications
- Pregnancy. Discuss with clinic if patient wishes to breast feed
- Severe renal or hepatic disease
- History of blood dyscrasia or exfoliative dermatitis

Table 3 Effect of auranofin on progression of radiological erosions

Reference	Comparator Drug	Duration	Result
Gofton et al. 1984	Placebo	12 months	Reduction in progression of erosions with auranofin compared with placebo
Capell et al. 1986	Placebo or GST	3 years	No difference between the three groups
Rau 1990	GST	3 years	Greater reduction in progression of erosions with GST compared with auranofin
Borg et al. 1991	Placebo	2 years	Reduction in progression of erosions with auranofin compared with placebo
Lopez-Mendez 1993	MTX or MTX plus auranofin	48 weeks	Significant progression of erosions seen only with auranofin alone
Weinblatt et al. 1993	MTX	36 weeks	Greater reduction in progression of erosions with MTX compared with auranofin
Prete et al. 1994	GST	24 months	Greater reduction in progression of erosions with aurothioglucose compared with auranofin
Glennas et al. 1997	Placebo	2 years	No difference between groups but relatively little deterioration in either

Gastrointestinal

Diarrhoea or loose stools is the commonest adverse event in most series occurring in up to 40–50% of patients with frank watery diarrhoea in 2–5% and, as with other gold-containing drugs, an ulcerative enterocolitis might very rarely occur. The mechanism of diarrhoea seems to be due to altered resorption of water and solutes by the colon. Diarrhoea usually responds to dosage reduction, bulking agents or temporary withdrawal, but in about 5% it may be severe enough to result in withdrawal of treatment.

Mucocutaneous

Mouth ulcers or rash, with or without pruritus, are common with rash occurring in up to 20%. In most cases this is mild and does not necessitate treatment withdrawal. However, occasionally this may be severe and the rash may be exfoliative. Up to 7% of patients may stop because of rash (Glennas et al. 1997; Gofton et al. 1984) although this may occur less often than with placebo (Glennas et al. 1997). The incidence of rash is approximately 50% of that seen with injectable gold salts (Scattenkirchner et al. 1988).

Proteinuria

About 3–5% of auranofin-treated patients develop persistent proteinuria resulting in treatment withdrawal. In the vast majority this resolves within 12 months and often does not recur on rechallenge.

■ BLOOD DYSCRASIAS

Auranofin may lead to thrombocytopenia and/or granulocytopenia. This is rare, but treatment should be discontinued. The decision to resume treatment (with close haematological monitoring) depends upon the clinical and laboratory pattern, which will indicate whether this was a true adverse effect.

HOW TO PRESCRIBE

- Provide patient and family doctor with written information about dose, therapeutic expectations, toxicity, monitoring requirements and action to take.
- Prescribe an initial dose of 3 mg BD changing if tolerated to 6 mg OD. After 6 months this can be increased to 9 mg daily (3 mg TID).
- Suggest a bulking agent if diarrhoea occurs.
- Supply a monitoring card for blood and urine and ensure that the patient is aware of the long-acting nature of the drug and the need for good compliance and regular monitoring.

■ TOXICITY MONITORING DURING AURANOFIN TREATMENT

As with most DMARDs most toxicity is concentrated within the first 6–12 months of treatment. The following protocol is suggested:

At baseline
- FBC, U&Es, LFTs, urinalysis, chest X-ray
- Education of patient with provision of written information and monitoring card, and dose and monitoring schedule for general practitioner

cont.

> *Regular monitoring*
> ■ Monthly FBC and urinalysis
>
> Patients should be advised to report rash, pruritus, mouth ulcers, bruising or abnormal bleeding.

Conception, pregnancy and lactation

Although data with auranofin are sparse, the manufacturers recommend that auranofin should be avoided in women during and for six months before pregnancy and that it should be avoided in breast-feeding mothers.

CONTRAINDICATIONS/CAUTIONS

■ Serious toxicity with other gold compounds
■ Pregnancy and lactation
■ Renal impairment or hepatic dysfunction
■ SLE (although there are some reports of its use in SLE)

Drug interactions

There are no specific interactions reported with auranofin but it would seem appropriate to avoid co-administration with chelating agents.

SUMMARY

Patients selected for auranofin:

■ Should have active inflammatory RA but perhaps those with more active disease should be considered for one of the more effective DMARDs
■ May be adults of any age
■ May have any disease duration

KEY REFERENCES

■ Wenger *et al.* 1983

■ Borg *et al.* 1988

■ Lopez-Mendez *et al.* 1993

■ Felson *et al.* 1991

■ McEntegart *et al.* 1996

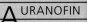

■ AURANOFIN—GP INFORMATION SHEET

Prescribing
Dosage: 3 mg bd increasing to 3 mg tid after 4–6 months if necessary

Monitoring
Pretreatment assessment: FBC, U&Es, LFTs, urinalysis

Monitoring: Monthly FBC and urinalysis. At each visit, patient should be asked about the presence of rash or oral ulceration

Please note that in addition to absolute values for haematological indices a rapid fall or a consistent downward trend in any value should prompt caution and extra vigilance.

Action to be taken if:

WBC $< 4.0 \times 10^9$/L	withhold *until discussed* with rheumatologist
Neutrophils $< 2.0 \times 10^9$/L	"　　"　　"　　"　　"
Platelets $< 150 \times 10^9$/L	"　　"　　"　　"　　"
$\geq$1+ proteinuria on >1 occasion	"　　"　　"　　"　　"
Rash or oral ulceration	"　　"　　"　　"　　"
Diarrhoea	increase fibre content of diet or add fibre supplements. May need to reduce dose or if severe stop treatment
Abnormal bruising or sore throat	withhold until FBC result available

Patient advice   The expected benefits and potential toxicity have been explained to your patient.

■ AURANOFIN (RIDAURA®)—(ORAL GOLD TABLETS)–PATIENT INFORMATION SHEET

Tablet size: 3 mg size tablets.

Dosage: Usually one tablet twice daily.

What does it do? It "dampens down" the inflammation in arthritic joints. The tablets are probably not as strong as gold injections, but on the other hand are less likely to cause side-effects.

Who needs treatment with auranofin?
It is reserved for use in patients who do not repond well enough to simpler treatment. It is used in RHEUMATOID ARTHRITIS and occasionally other less common forms of arthritis.

What benefit can be expected?
The drug may take up to 6 months (usually quicker) before the joint symptoms start to improve. Treatment with other arthritis medication is usually continued.

What are the possible side-effects?
- Some looseness of the bowels is noticed by many patients but is usually not serious and tends to subside after a few weeks of treatment.
- Skin reactions such as itching or rash may occur. If the reaction is mild, treatment may be continued after adjustment of dosage (but consult your doctor).
- Mouth ulcers or soreness of tongue and mouth (stomatitis).
- Reduction in the white blood cell or platelet count may occur and this may mean that treatment must be stopped. These changes may lead to infection or bleeding.
- Irritation of the kidney leading to the appearance of protein in the urine. THE RISK OF EACH OF THESE SIDE-EFFECTS IS MINIMIZED BY FOLLOWING THE PRECAUTIONS DESCRIBED BELOW.

What precautions are necessary?
1. Report anything that you suspect may be a side-effect to your doctor. Ensure that you tell your doctor about any previous side-effects to other medicines.
2. Report to the doctor urgently if you develop any of the following:
   Abnormal bleeding tendency (excessive bruising, blood spots or blisters on the skin or in the mouth).
   Severe sore throat.
   Generalized itching, rash, mouth ulcers or soreness of the mouth.
3. A monthly blood and urine test is required to ensure that the blood count is normal and that the kidneys are not being irritated. The frequency of these tests will be determined by your specialist.

IF THERE IS ANYTHING ELSE YOU WISH TO KNOW, PLEASE DO NOT HESITATE TO ASK

3 DMARDs

PENICILLAMINE

KEY INDICATIONS

- Rheumatoid arthritis

■ INTRODUCTION

Penicillamine along with intramuscular (IM) gold was one of the earliest disease-modifying antirheumatic drugs (DMARDs) regularly used to treat rheumatoid arthritis. The position of penicillamine in the therapeutic ladder has declined as other agents such as sulphasalazine (SASP), methotrexate and leflunomide have shown a better efficacy/toxicity profile. Nevertheless, penicillamine remains a useful drug when other treatments are no longer an option.

■ PHARMACOLOGY

Penicillamine is an amino acid with a thiol side chain. There are two enantiomers but only the D type is of clinical interest. Oral absorption is excellent with a bioavalibility of 40–70% in fasted subjects. Bioavailability is markedly reduced if the dose is taken with food, antacids or iron supplements.

On absorption penicillamine is rapidly oxidized and forms a variety of disulphides including disulphides with itself. The serum half-life is 2–4 hours after a single dose, this rises to 4–6 days with regular therapy. Clearance of the disulphides is mainly in the urine.

■ BENEFIT

Most studies investigating penicillamine were performed before 1985 and included relatively small numbers of patients. These studies preceded the widespread use of currently recognized composite scores of efficacy such as the ACR response rate and the DAS.

■ MONOTHERAPY

There have been four randomized placebo-controlled studies of sufficient size using penicillamine in the treatment of rheumatoid arthritis and these are summarized in Table 1. Doses of penicillamine used varied from 125 mg/day to 1500 mg/day. There was a higher dropout rate due to side-effects in groups on doses in excess of 1000 mg. There were improvements in a number of clinical and laboratory parameters in each of the studies including duration of morning stiffness (reduced by ~80%), pain and articular index of joint tenderness (reduced by ~ 50%), erythrocyte sedimentation rate (ESR) reduced by 34% and also significant improvements in patient and physician assessments. Withdrawal rates at six months for doses between 500 and 600 mg/day were 29–34%.

There have been comparative studies of penicillamine against azathioprine, SASP, hydroxychloroquine (HCQ), oral and IM gold, and these are summarized in Table 2. Penicillamine was found to be better than HCQ and oral gold. There was no difference in efficacy between penicillamine and any of the other agents. These findings have been reinforced in a meta-analysis undertaken by Felson *et al.*, which showed penicillamine to have similar efficacy to SASP, IM gold and methotrexate and to be more effective than oral gold.

■ LONG-TERM STUDIES

There are very few studies of penicillamine therapy over a five-year period. Approximately one-fifth of patients remain on therapy after this period, with most stopping because of side-effects. One open randomized study found that 53% of patients continued penicillamine at five years. This may have been due to the low mean daily dose (396 mg). Nevertheless, in this study significantly more patients remained on penicillamine than on HCQ or oral or injectable gold.

■ COMBINATION THERAPY

Penicillamine has been tried in combination with a number of other agents. These have included SASP, IM gold, HCQ and azathioprine. There is no good published evidence to suggest that any of these combinations are superior to penicillamine alone, and therefore combination therapy with penicillamine is not recommended.

■ RADIOLOGICAL PROGRESSION

No substantial studies have been performed with penicillamine in which radiological progression has been a primary endpoint. One small study comparing penicillamine to HCQ found less radiological progression in the penicillamine group at 12 months. The difference between the groups at two years was no longer significant.

Table 1 Randomized placebo controlled studies

	Year	No. of patients	Groups	Max. daily dose	Study duration (weeks)	Comments
Multi-centre Trials group	1973	105	2	1500 mg	52	High dose with high withdrawals
Dixon et al.	1975	121	3	600/1200 mg	24	Efficacy similar at both doses and >placebo
Shiokawa et al.	1977	179	2	600 mg	24	44% response at 12 weeks 65% at 24 weeks
Williams et al.	1983	225	3	125/500 mg	30	Lower dose no better than placebo

Table 2 Comparative studies

Author	Year	Comparator drug	No. in study	Result
Hochberg	1986	Auranofin	88	D-penicillamine >efficacy and toxicity
Gibson et al.	1976	Myocrisin	87	No difference
Thomas et al.	1984	Myocrisin	50	No difference
Bunch et al.	1984	HCQ/comb	54	D-penicillamine >efficacy
Capell et al.	1990	SASP	200	No difference
Paulus et al.	1984	Azathioprine	206	No difference
Berry et al.	1976	Azathioprine	65	No difference

EFFICACY

- Penicillamine is an effective drug for the clinical features of active rheumatoid arthritis.
- The efficacy of penicillamine is similar to that of methotrexate, sulphasalazine, IM gold and azathioprine.
- Penicillamine is more effective than auranofin and hydroxychloroquine.
- Toxicity is the commonest cause for withdrawal.

■ TOXICITY

Adverse reactions will lead to withdrawal of penicillamine in approximately 20–30% of individuals within a year. Toxicity is more common at higher doses. The most important adverse reactions are shown in Table 3. There does not appear to be any evidence for cumulative toxicity, although serious side-effects can occur at any time during penicillamine therapy and thus continued monitoring of patients is essential.

In a 12-year follow-up study of 98 patients sustained improvement in inflammatory parameters was seen. No drug-related deaths occurred. Proteinuria (17%), thrombocytopenia (4%), rash (9%) and mouth ulcers (4%) all reversed on stopping therapy. One late case of drug-induced systemic lupus erythematosus (SLE) was observed. There were no deaths attributed to penicillamine.

Table 3 Management of toxicity

Adverse event	Occurrence rate	Clinical management
Mucocutaneous Mouth ulcers, urticarial rashes, pruritus, lichen planus	10–20	Withhold penicillamine and consider alternative causes. If reaction mild then cautiously re-introduce at a lower dose. Beware of pemphigus rash, which requires immediate and permanent treatment cessation
Pemphigus	Rare	Stop Rx
Gastrointestinal Dysgeusia and nausea	10–20	Reassure that this is that it usually a temporary phenomenon. Explain will settle over 4–6 weeks. Dose reduction may be necessary
Renal Proteinuria (trace) Proteinuria (+ or more)	5–10	Continue therapy. If confirmed on repeat testing then perform 24-hour collection. If >1 g/24 hours then stop penicillamine. If <1 g then therapy can continue with monitoring of proteinuria.
Haematuria		In absence of proteinuria and with normal renal function penicillamine can be continued while other potential causes are investigated. If no cause found consider discontinuing penicillamine.
Glomerulonephritis Goodpasture's syndrome	Rare	Stop therapy
Haematological Thrombocytopenia <150 × 10⁹/L.	1–4%	Reduce dose. May need to stop Rx. If gradual and mild then stop penicillamine till platelet count normalises and consider gradual re-introduction at a lower dose with close monitoring. If precipitous then stop treatment permanently.
Leucopenia and aplastic anaemia Fall in WBC <4 × 10⁹ or neutrophils <2 × 10⁹	Very rare	Stop therapy
Abnormal LFTs	Rare	Stop Rx
Lungs Bronchiolitis obliterans	Rare	Stop Rx
Immunological SLE, myasthenia gravis, polymyositis	Rare	Stop Rx

■ GASTROINTESTINAL

Dysgeusia (altered taste) is an important adverse effect that can occur early in therapy. Patients should be reassured that this is usually a temporary phenomenon and usually resolves without intervention. In a small number it may persist necessitating cessation of treatment. Significant nausea and bowel upset are rare with penicillamine.

■ MUCOCUTANEOUS

Mucocutaneous reactions are the commonest side-effect of penicillamine and can lead to withdrawal in 10–20% of cases. Mouth ulcers may occur in a dose-dependent manner and a dose reduction can lead to resolution without having to discontinue therapy. Mild skin eruptions can be managed similarly. A pemphigus-like rash, however, requires immediate and permanent cessation of treatment.

■ HAEMATOLOGICAL

Haematological reactions are the commonest cause of death secondary to penicillamine recorded by the Committee on Safety of Medicines. The fatalities are generally due to neutropenia or marrow aplasia. A fall in the total white blood count to $< 4.0 \times 10^9$ or of neutrophils to $< 2 \times 10^9$ should lead to immediate discontinuation of penicillamine and, if confirmed, penicillamine should not be reintroduced.

Thrombocytopenia
Thrombocytopenia is more common than leucopenia and appears to be dose related. It is thought to be due to a direct toxic effect on megakaryocytes. If the fall is gradual and the thrombocytopenia mild then penicillamine can often be restarted at a lower dose with careful monitoring of the platelet count. If the fall is sudden and precipitous then penicillamine should be withheld permanently. An isolated fall in haemoglobin with other blood constituents being normal is unlikely to be due to penicillamine, and other causes should be considered.

■ RENAL

Penicillamine can lead to an immune complex-mediated glomerulonephritis. This gives rise to proteinuria, which can be detected using dipstix analysis. If a value of one + or more is detected on two occasions then a 24-hour estimation of urinary protein loss should be undertaken. If this confirms excretion of $< 1\,\text{g}$

then penicillamine should be withheld. A study of 33 patients found that the proteinuria resolved in all cases, although this took up to 21 months. Another small study found that it was possible to re-introduce penicillamine at a lower dose without recurrence. Haematuria is rare with penicillamine and other causes should be considered whilst penicillamine is withheld. Goodpasture's syndrome has been reported as a side-effect of penicillamine

■ PULMONARY

Bronchiolitis obliterans has been reported with penicillamine and also, as mentioned above, very rarely Goodpasture's syndrome.

■ AUTOIMMUNE

A number of autoimmune conditions have been reported in association with penicillamine treatment. These include: polymyositis, myasthenia gravis, SLE and Goodpasture's syndrome.

■ MISCELLANEOUS

Mammary hyperplasia has been reported in both males and females.

■ DRUG INTERACTIONS

Penicillamine is a chelating agent and will bind to iron and constituents of antacids, reducing the effective dose of penicillamine. Therefore, these agents should be taken at least two hours after penicillamine. No other clinically relevant drug interactions have been reported.

■ PREGNANCY AND LACTATION

Penicillamine will cause fetal connective tissue abnormalities in 5% of pregnancies. Women of child-bearing potential should be advised to use adequate contraception and to stop penicillamine immediately if they become pregnant. It is our practice to recommend stopping penicillamine three months before attempted conception.

There are no data on the excretion of penicillamine in breast milk; however, penicillamine should probably be avoided by breast-feeding mothers.

■ MONITORING

Regular monitoring is required to minimize the risk of significant toxicity with penicillamine. Guidelines have been proposed by the British Society for Rheumatology (BSR) and are outlined below.

BSR guidelines for penicillamine monitoring	
FBC	Baseline then every 2 weeks until a stable dose then 4 weekly
Urinalysis	Baseline then every 2 weeks until a stable dose then 4 weekly
U&Es and creatinine	Baseline

■ Patients should be supplied with a drug information sheet and monitoring card and advised to discontinue penicillamine and attend their doctor if they develop a sore throat, bleeding or abnormal bruising.

PRACTICAL PRESCRIBING

- ■ **Counselling:** The use of penicillamine should be discussed with the patient. The benefits, potential toxicity and monitoring schedule should be outlined verbally and reinforced with a written information sheet.

- ■ **Dosage**: Therapy should be started at a dose of 125 mg daily taken first thing in the morning on an empty stomach.
- ■ The dose is increased at 4-weekly intervals until a response is achieved or 500 mg daily is being taken.
- ■ Penicillamine may take 3–6 months to become effective.
- ■ If after 6 months an adequate clinical response has not been achieved, the dose can be increased to 750 mg for 12 weeks and then to 1 g by similar increments for a further 12 weeks.
- ■ Lack of response at this dose suggests that penicillamine is unlikely to be effective and that treatment should be discontinued.

- ■ **Cautions**: Caution is required in the presence of significant renal impairment.

- ■ **Contraindications**: Penicillamine should be avoided in patients with RA/connective tissue disease overlap syndromes. Penicillamine should not be used during pregnancy or breast feeding.

Management of toxicity

See Table 3 on p. 95.

SUMMARY

- Penicillamine is an effective treatment for the clinical features of active rheumatoid arthritis
- There is no good evidence that it can retard radiological progression
- Penicillamine should only be used after drugs with a similar efficacy but better toxicity profile (e.g. methotrexate, sulphasalazine and leflunomide)
- Penicillamine toxicity can be minimized by using the smallest effective dose, regular monitoring and awareness of its side-effect profile

---

KEY REFERENCES

- Multi-centre Trial Group 1973

- Gibson *et al.* 1976

- Capell *et al.* 1990

- Munro *et al.* 1997

- Jessop *et al.* 1998

■ PENICILLAMINE—GP INFORMATION SHEET

Penicillamine is used to treat rheumatoid arthritis. Toxicity can occur, but if certain precautions are taken, most patients tolerate penicillamine without serious problems. It may take 12–24 weeks before an effect is seen.

Prescribing
- The usual starting dose is 125 mg daily
- The usual increase in daily dose is 125 mg every 4 weeks, until a response is seen or 500 mg daily is achieved. If after 6 months no effect is seen the dose can be increased to 750 mg by increments of 125 mg/4-weekly for 12 weeks then 1000 mg by similar increments for a further 12 weeks.
- Penicillamine should be taken first thing in the morning on an empty stomach at least 30 minutes before food

Patients will still need their NSAID and analgestic drugs, although these can sometimes by stopped/reduced if/when the patient responds to penicillamine

Absolute contraindications   Pregnancy or planned pregnancy, RA/SLE overlap syndromes

Cautions   Renal impairment

Drug interactions   Iron supplements and antacids should be taken at least 2 hours after penicillamine

Blood monitoring
We would be grateful for your help in monitoring this therapy. We suggest:
- FBC/diff—fortnightly until dose is stable, thereafter every 4 weeks
- Urinalysis—fortnightly until dose is stable, thereafter every 4 weeks

Management of toxicity: see below

Side-effect	Action
Mucocutaneous reaction	Withhold penicillamine and consider alternative causes. If reaction mild then cautiously re-introduce at a lower dose. Beware of pemphigus rash which requires immediate and permanent treatment cessation.
Loss of taste/dysgeusia	Reassure that this is usually a temporary phenomenon.
White cell count $< 4 \times 10^9$/L, PMN <2	Stop penicillamine and contact rheumatology unit.
Platelet count $< 150 \times 10^9$/L	Stop penicillamine and contact rheumatology unit.
Haemoglobin <9 g/dL	Check haematinics and contact rheumatology unit.
Proteinuria (trace)	Continue therapy.
Proteinuria (+ or more)	If confirmed on two occasions then stop penicillamine and contact rheumatology unit.
Haematuria	If confirmed on two occasions discuss with rheumatology unit.

Patient advice   The patients have been given an information sheet about the expected benefits and potential side-effects of penicillamine therapy.

3 DMARDs

L EFLUNOMIDE

KEY INDICATIONS

- Adult patients with active rheumatoid arthritis

■ INTRODUCTION

Leflunomide is a new disease-modifying antirheumatic drug (DMARD) for rheumatoid arthritis (RA) with a more rapid onset of action and a comparable efficacy and toxicity profile to that of methotrexate and sulphasalazine.

■ PHARMACOLOGY

Mode of action

Leflunomide is an isoxazole derivative rapidly converted by first-pass metabolism in the gut and liver to its active metabolite. It is 99% protein bound in plasma, and is excreted in equal proportions in urine and faeces. It has a long half-life of between one and four weeks. Benefit is thought to be due to inhibition of dihydro-orotate dehydrogenase, a key enzyme in the pyrimidine synthesis pathway utilized by rapidly dividing cells such as activated T-cells. Other immunomodulatory effects include blockade of tumour necrosis factor-mediated activation of the transcription factor NFκB of leucocyte migration and chemotaxis. Generations of reactive oxygen radicals and matrix metalloproteinases are also inhibited.

■ BENEFIT

Efficacy in RA

Three double-blind randomized controlled trials of leflunomide provide the core evidence base for benefit in RA (see Table 1). The methotrexate study reported by Strand et al. (1999) was extended for a further 12 months, omitting the placebo arm (Cohen et al. 2001).

Table 1 Leflunomide (LEF) in rheumatoid comparative studies

Reference	n	Comparative drugs	Study design/ disease duration	Duration of follow-up	Outcome efficacy	Outcome toxicity	Conclusion/ comment
Scott et al. 2001	358	LEF/SASP/ placebo	DBPCRT—6 months Placebo arm switched to SASP at 6 months for rest of study. 5–8 years disease duration	24 months	LEF and SASP significantly better than placebo. LEF superior to SASP at 24 months for HAQ, global scores, ACR 20 and 50 response rates.	Fewer adverse events at 6, 12, 24 months with LEF cf. SASP.	LEF efficacious, safe and better than SASP for certain outcome measures
Strand et al. 1999	482	LEF/MTX/ placebo	DBPCRT 6.7 years disease duration	12 months	LEF and MTX significantly better than placebo. LEF more effective than MTX at improving HAQ- delaying radiographic progression.	22% LEF vs 10% MTX withdrawals due to AEs. Serious AEs fewer on LEF, however	Efficacy shown. Some advantages of LEF over MTX. All patients on folic acid

Emery et al. 2000	999	LEF/MTX	DBRT 3.5–3.8 years disease duration	24 months	3 of 4 primary outcome measures significantly better with MTX cf. LEF at 1 year. Differences in efficacy less at 2 years	19% LEF vs 15% MTX withdrawals due to AEs at 1 year. Serious AEs 7% LEF vs 8% MTX. 2 deaths in MTX group, none on LEF. Hepatotoxicity 3-fold higher with MTX than LEF	Folic acid <10%
Cohen et al. 2001	199	LEF/MTX	DBRT 5.9–6.7 years disease duration	12 month extension of Strand et al. 1999 (placebo arm dropped)	ACR response/ radiographic changes same for LEF + MTX. LEF had significant benefit on HAQ cf MTX	Toxicity profile same over year 2 as year 1	LEF equivalent to MTX all measures better for HAQ

Study 1 Scott *et al.* (2001) compared leflunomide with sulphasalazine (SASP) and placebo in 358 patients. At 6 months patients in the placebo arm of the study were switched to SASP, and follow-up continued to 24 months (see Figure 1). Leflunomide demonstrated significant benefit over placebo in all clinical and laboratory measures of activity function and radiological progression. ACR 20, 50 and 70 response rates for leflunomide and SASP were similar at 6 months (see Table 2) and improvement was maintained at 12 months.

Table 2 Percentage of patients achieving ACR response criteria. Leflunomide vs SASP vs placebo (6-month data)

	Leflunomide	SASP	Placebo	NNT
ACR 20 response	55%	56%	29%	4
ACR 50 response	33%	30%	14%	5

Study 2 The Leflunomide RA Investigators Group compared leflunomide, placebo and methotrexate in 485 patients over 12 months (Strand *et al.* 1999). All patients were on 1 mg of folate once or twice daily. Leflunomide was better than placebo in all components of the ACR response (Table 3). ACR response rates were equivalent to those for patients receiving methotrexate. Leflunomide-treated patients had a greater improvement in HAQ score (–0.45 vs –0.26, $p < 0.01$) compared to patients in the methotrexate group. Radiographic progression on leflunomide was less than on methotrexate and just reached statistical significance—change in Sharp score at 12 months for patients on leflunomide compared with those on methotrexate (0.53 vs 0.88, $p = 0.05$).

Table 3 Percentage of patients achieving ACR response criteria. Leflunomide RA Investigators Group Study. Leflunomide vs MTX, 12-month data

	Leflunomide	MTX	Placebo	NNT*
ACR 20 response	52%	46%	26%	4
ACR 50 response	34%	23%	8%	4
ACR 70 response	20%	9%	4%	6

* NNT, number-needed-to-treat to gain are additional responders with leflunomide compared with placebo.

Study 3 Emery *et al.* (2000) observed an ACR 20 response rate at 12 months of 50% with leflunomide and 65% with methotrexate. Methotrexate provided more benefit than leflunomide in swollen joint count, physician global score and patient global score at one year, but by two years the differences

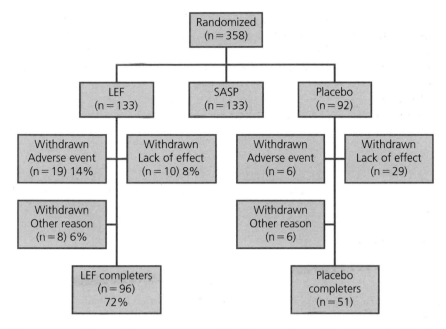

Figure 1 Leflunomide vs SASP vs placebo. Study results for 0–6 months. *(Smolen et al. 1999)*

between the two treatment groups were no longer apparent. In this study, < 10% of patients were on folic acid therapy. Folic acid supplementation while reducing toxicity from methotrexate may also lead to a reduction in efficacy (Smolen *et al.* 1999). This may explain the greater response to methotrexate in this study. The ACR 20 response to leflunomide is strikingly similar in both studies.

Radiographic benefit from leflunomide
Leflunomide delays radiographic progression significantly compared to placebo. Leflunomide showed significant benefit over placebo at 6 months using the Larsen score (see Table 4). Patients followed-up to 24 months on leflunomide had a reduction in Larsen score from 1.48 (±0.65) at baseline to 1.38 (±0.59) (Larsen *et al.* 2001).

Table 4 Radiographic benefit of leflunomide compared to placebo using the Larsen score means and standard deviations.

	Leflunomide	Placebo
Baseline Larsen score	1.48 (0.65)	1.49 (0.60)
Increase in Larsen score at 6 months	0.01 (0.03)*	0.05 (0.09)
*p<0.05 vs placebo.		

Table 5   Radiographic benefit of leflunomide compared to placebo using the Sharp score. Mean (SD) shown.

	Leflunomide (n = 131)	Placebo (n = 83)
Baseline Sharp score	23.11 (34.0)	25.37 (31.3)
Increase in Sharp score at 1 year	0.53 (4.5)*	2.16 (4.0)

*p ≤ 0.001 vs placebo.

When X-rays were read using the Sharp method, Strand *et al.* (1999) demonstrated a significant reduction in radiographic progression at one year (see Table 5).

Long-term follow-up
This is not yet available for leflunomide. Response has been shown to be maintained to 24 months.

Combination therapy
Leflunomide has been used in combination with methotrexate, sulphasalazine and infliximab.

- Increased hepatotoxicity was reported with methotrexate.
- In a retrospective cohort study of 93 patients on leflunomide and infliximab there was one death from acute respiratory distress syndrome/pneumonia.
- Leflunomide in combination with sulphasalazine appeared to be well tolerated, with no convincing benefit over monotherapy.

■ EVIDENCE FOR HARM

Adverse events on leflunomide which have required withdrawal for studies are less than on SASP but more often than with methotrexate. Potential side-effects of leflunomide are outlined below. Diarrhoea, nausea and alopecia are common (see Table 6).

Serious adverse events
No lefunomide- or SASP-related deaths occurred during the studies, but there were three deaths directly attributed to methotrexate therapy—one from pneumonitis, and two from sepsis (one secondary to pancytopenia).

Haematological toxicity
Of leflunomide treated-patients in one study (van Ede *et al.* 1999), 0.8% developed leucopenia requiring treatment discontinuation.

Table 6 Potential toxicity of leflunomide

Adverse event	Frequency	Action
Gastrointestinal Nausea Diarrhoea Abdominal pain	Common	Antiemetic Consider dose reduction
Abnormal LFTs	Common	<3 fold increase, reduce to 10 mg/day. >3 fold increase, stop leflunomide
Alopecia	Common	Dose reduction initially. Stop if severe
Skin rash	Common	Dose reduction or stop if severe.
Hypertension	Common	Usually mild increase. Often pre-existing high blood pressure
Haematological Leucopenia Neutropenia Anaemia Thrombocytopenia	Uncommon	Stop therapy if: WBC $< 4 \times 10^9/l$ Neutrophils $< 2 \times 10^9/L$ Platelets $< 150 \times 10^9/L$
Jaundice/ hepatic failure	Very rare	Stop therapy. Can be fatal

Common	1–10% of patients
Uncommon	0.1–1%
Rare	0.01–0.1%
Very rare	0.01%

Hepatotoxicity

Emery *et al.* (2000) reported three-fold greater hepatotoxicity with methotrexate than with leflunomide. This may, in part, be attributable to the lack of folic acid supplementation in this study.

■ PRACTICAL PRESCRIBING

HOW TO PRESCRIBE LEFLUNOMIDE

- Leflunomide is available in 10, 20 and 100 mg tablets.
- Check baseline FBC, LFTs and blood pressure.
- Give loading dose: 100 mg /day for three days.
- Maintenance dose thereafter: 20 mg /day.
- NSAIDs and analgesics should be continued as usual.
- Provide patient information and a monitoring card.
- Dose reduction to 10 mg /day can be used if patient develops minor side-effects.

CAUTIONS

- Male and female patients should be advised about the use of contraception while on leflunomide, and for at least two years after treatment in women and three months after treatment in men.
- Vaccination with live vaccines is not recommended.

CONTRAINDICATIONS

- Pregnant women, women of child-bearing age not using contraception, breast-feeding mothers
- Impaired liver function
- Severe immunodeficiency, bone marrow suppression or serious infections
- Moderate or severe renal impairment
- Severe hypoproteinaemia (e.g. nephrotic syndrome)

GUIDELINES FOR MONITORING LEFLUNOMIDE RX

At baseline
- FBC, urea & electrolytes, liver function tests, blood pressure
- Education of patient, provision of monitoring card, written information to patient, shared care protocol to primary care provider

cont.

During initiation of RX
- Fortnightly FBC and biochemistry for 24 weeks then every 8 weeks.

Long term
- 8-weekly

Reinforce advice about long half-life and washout procedure necessary if pregnancy planned. Pregnancy test at baseline may be necessary.

PREGNANCY

The active metabolite of leflunomide is teratogenic in animals. The manufacturers recommend performing a pregnancy test prior to starting treatment. A reliable method of contraception must be used throughout the treatment period. Female patients are advised to wait two years after stopping treatment with leflunomide before conceiving. If this is not possible a washout procedure with cholestyramine or activated charcoal is advised (see below). Thereafter plasma concentrations of the active drug should be <0.02 mg/L on two occasions 14 days apart and the patient should wait one and a half months after the first plasma concentration of <0.02 mg/L before conception. Both cholestyramine and activated charcoal can interfere with the effectiveness of the oral contraceptive pill.

BREAST FEEDING

Leflunomide is found in breast milk in animal studies. It should therefore be avoided during breast feeding.

MALE FERTILITY

No data are available on potential fetal toxicity. Contraception while on leflunomide is advised. If pregnancy is planned, males should be advised to stop leflunomide and wait three months. If two plasma levels of active matobolate 14 days apart are <0.02 mg/L the risk of fetal toxicity is very low.

DRUG INTERACTIONS

- Caution is advised with the concentrated use of cytochrome P450 metabolized drugs (phenytoin, warfarin, tolbutamide).
- With other DMARDs, co-administration with methotrexate may lead to increased hepatotoxicity.
- Rifampicin increases the levels of leflunomide by 40%.
- ?should avoid live vaccines.

WASHOUT PROCEDURE IF REQUIRED

- Cholestyramine 8 g TID for 11 days.
  or
- Activated charcoal 50 g QID for 11 days.

SUMMARY

- Leflunomide is a relatively new DMARD of proven efficacy for RA.
- The long half-life has important implications for pregnancy planning and management of major toxicity.

KEY REFERENCES

- Scott *et al.* 2001

- Strand *et al.* 1999

- Emery *et al.* 2000

- Cohen *et al.* 2001

- Smolen *et al.* 1999

■ LEFLUNOMIDE—GP INFORMATION SHEET

Effect
Leflunomide is a new immunomodulatory agent which has been shown to be effective as a disease modifying agent in rheumatoid arthritis (RA). It has a fairly rapid onset of action. Benefits may be apparent as early as 4 weeks after starting therapy and further improvement may be seen up to 4–6 months.

Prescribing
An initial loading dose of 100 mg per day for 3 days is followed by a maintenance of 20 mg daily. NSAIDs and analgesics should be continued, although these may be reduced or stopped if the patient responds to leflunomide.

Monitoring
Baseline FBC and LFTs will be checked at the rheumatology clinic. Thereafter, the patient should have blood checks every 2 weeks for the first 6 months and then every 8 weeks thereafter. Please ensure the results are entered on the patient-held monitoring card. Blood pressure should be monitored at each check.

Contraindications/fertility
Leflunomide is contraindicated in pregnancy or breast-feeding mothers. The manufacturers recommend that 2 years should elapse after cessation of therapy before elective pregnancy.

Cautions
- Not recommended in patients with severe immunodeficiency, bone marrow dysplasia or severe uncontrolled infections.
- Vaccination with live vaccines not recommended.
- Use with caution in patients with renal impairment or if the patient is taking rifampicin. Drugs which inhibit cytochrome P450 such as phenytoin or warfarin will need further monitoring.
- Use other potentially hepatotoxic medications with caution.
- Alcohol should be avoided.

Toxicity
Leflunomide is generally well tolerated. Commonest side-effects are nausea, diarrhoea, skin rashes, alopecia and mild increase in blood pressure. Rarely, neutropenia or abnormalities of LFTs have been

cont.

observed. Side-effects usually respond to dose reduction or reverse on drug discontinuation, but may take several weeks because of the long half-life. Mild elevations in blood pressure have been noted, particularly in those with pre-existing hypertension.

Adverse effect management

Nausea: Try antiemetic or reduce dose

Rash: Try dose reduction or stop if severe

Alopecia: Try dose reduction initially

Neutropenia: Stop therapy and contact rheumatology unit

Abnormal LFTs: If >2 but <3 fold increase above normal range, reduce dose to 10 mg/day
                 If >3 fold increase above normal range, stop and contact GRI

Washout procedure

Cholestyramine or activated powdered charcoal can be used if washout is considered necessary. Please contact CRD.

Patient advice   The expected benefits and potential toxicity have been explained to your patient.

3 DMARDs

MINOCYCLINE

KEY INDICATIONS

- Rheumatoid arthritis (not licensed)

■ INTRODUCTION

There is interest in the concept that the aetiology of rheumatoid arthritis (RA) may be infectious. While this remains contentious, it has resulted in the serendipitous discovery of various effective disease-modifying antirheumatic drugs (DMARDs) including sulphasalazine, gold, hydroxychloroquine and, most recently, minocycline. There is now a core of good evidence that minocycline is of benefit in controlling disease activity in RA, particularly in early disease. No trials have been undertaken in other forms of inflammatory arthritis. The routine use of minocycline in RA remains rather limited, largely due to the dearth of published data relative to other established DMARDs.

■ PHARMACOLOGY

The tetracyclines are antibiotics that are thought to exert their bacteriostatic effects by inhibiting bacterial protein synthesis. Minocycline is a semisynthetic derivative of tetracycline. Minocycline hydrochloride is readily absorbed orally and peak serum levels are attained after 1–4 hours. The drug is primarily renally excreted.

Possible mechanisms of action of minocycline in RA include inhibition of matrix metalloproteinases, inhibition of inducible nitric oxide synthetase expression and inhibition of T-cell proliferation.

■ EFFICACY

- A number of uncontrolled, observational studies initially suggested a role for minocycline in RA.
- These findings have now been supported by three double-blind, randomized, placebo-controlled trials (Bluhm *et al.* 1997; Kloppenburg *et al.* 1994; O'Dell *et al.* 1997).

- In a recent trial, minocycline was shown to be more effective than hydroxychloroquine (O'Dell *et al.* 2001).
- Minocycline is thought to be less effective than mainstream DMARDs such as sulphasalazine and methotrexate, but no direct comparison has been made in a trial setting.

Clinical

The core evidence of benefit is from three double-blind randomized placebo-controlled trials and a comparative study with hydroxychloroquine. The first placebo-controlled trial performed demonstrated statistically significant improvements in the erythrocyte sedimentation rate (ESR) and the Ritchie articular index (Bluhm *et al.* 1997) over 26 weeks. A second trial showed significant improvements in both primary endpoints, namely 50% reduction in swollen and tender joint counts, over placebo (Kloppenburg *et al.* 1994). The first trial allowed use of concomitant DMARD therapy, whereas the second did not. These trials were performed in patients with relatively advanced disease with median disease durations of 13 and 8.5 years respectively.

In a placebo-controlled trial in early RA (defined as less than one year's duration), minocycline was better than placebo. A 50% improvement according to modified Paulus composite criteria was used as the primary endpoint (see Table 1).

Table 1	Primary endpoint results, minocycline vs placebo (O'Dell *et al.* 1997)		
	Minocycline 100 mg bd	*Placebo*	*p Value*
50% improvement (modified Paulus)	65%	13%	<0.001

Comparative studies

In a comparison of minocycline with hydroxychloroquine in patients with early disease on low-dose oral prednisolone, minocycline was superior (see Table 2).

Radiographic evidence

Only one study (Kloppenburg *et al.* 1994) analysed radiographic changes. The study was of short duration (one year) and not adequately powered to detect differences in radiographic outcomes. No statistical difference was demonstrated between minocycline and placebo for erosion progression rates or for joint space narrowing (Tilley *et al.* 1995). There was, however, a trend towards benefit in the treatment group in all parameters assessed.

Table 2 Clinical parameters at two years (O'Dell *et al.* 2001)

	Minocycline 100 mg bd	Hydoxychloroquine 200 mg bd	p Value
ACR 20	67%	43%	0.06
ACR 50*	60%	33%	0.04
ACR 70	43%	27%	0.14
Mean prednisolone dose at 2 years (mg)*	0.81	3.21	<0.01

*Primary endpoint, minocycline vs hydroxychloroquine.

■ HARM

Adverse reactions (see Table 3) are generally less common than with other DMARDs. It is particularly important to note that dizziness is a relatively common complaint which is of concern in frail, elderly patients. Skin pigmentation is relatively common and usually occurs after 18 months of therapy. It is often slate grey and can resemble bruising on extremities in early stages.

Table 3 Minocycline-related toxicity

	Adverse effect	Early/Late	Dose-related (DR)/ idiosyncratic (I)
Most common	GI upset (mainly nausea)	Early	DR
	Dizziness	Early	DR
	Skin pigmentation	Late	DR
	Maculopapular rash	Early	I
	Headache	Early	I
	Hepatitis	Early–Medium	DR
	Lupus syndrome	Early–Medium	I
	Blood dyscrasias (e.g. ↓ platelets)	Early–Medium	?
	Renal (↑ urea)	Early–Medium	?
	Benign intracranial hypertension	Early–Medium	I
Most rare	Stevens–Johnson syndrome	Early	I

■ PRESCRIBING

It is recommended that patients start on 50 mg bd for four weeks and increase to 100 mg bd thereafter, assuming no adverse effects. All of the published evidence for efficacy in RA relates to the standard 100 mg bd dosage. However, if patients develop side-effects they may revert to the lower starting dose.

GUIDELINES FOR MONITORING MINOCYCLINE IN RA

Blood monitoring
- Full blood count, urea and electrolytes and liver function tests should be checked at baseline and every three months while on therapy.
- Provide written information for patient and general practice.
- Be alert for pigmentation changes and possibly of drug-induced SLE.

Pregnancy, lactation and fertility
- Tetracyclines are teratogenic and should be stopped if pregnancy is suspected.
- Women of child-bearing age should be advised to take adequate steps to prevent conception.
- Minocycline may impair efficacy of oral contraceptives.
- Minocycline is excreted in human milk and, may cause damage to the developing child and nursing mothers should not be prescribed this drug.
- Studies in rats suggest that minocycline impairs male fertility but this finding is not supported by human data.

Drug interactions
Table 4 shows the major drug interactions with minocycline.

Table 4 Major drug interactions with minocycline

Drug	Interaction	Advice
Warfarin	Minocycline reduces prothrombin activity	Warfarin dose may need to be reduced
Oral contraceptive pill	Efficacy of pill may be impaired	Advise alternative means of contraception
Antacids Iron preparations	Impair absorption of minocycline	Avoid administration within 3 hours of each other
Penicillins	Minocycline may reduce efficacy of bactericidal effects	Avoid co-administration

CONTRAINDICATIONS

■ Pregnancy
■ Breast feeding
■ Children under 12 years
■ Renal impairment
■ Hepatic impairment

SUMMARY

■ Minocycline is a safe, well-tolerated drug that seems to be efficacious in reducing disease activity in RA.
■ It remains a useful option for patients who have failed to tolerate or respond to more established DMARDs.

KEY REFERENCES

■ Kloppenburg *et al.* 1994

■ Tilley *et al.* 1995

■ O'Dell *et al.* 1997

■ O'Dell *et al.* 2002

■ Bluhn *et al.* 1997

Table 5 Summary of the major trials of minocycline in rheumatoid arthritis

Reference	n	Comparator drug	Study design (disease duration)	Duration of follow-up	Efficacy	Toxicity	Conclusion
Kloppenburg et al. 1994	80	Placebo	Randomized, double-blind (median disease duration 13 years)	26 weeks	Significant improvement in lab parameters with minocycline; clinical improvement less pronounced	Largely GI toxicity and dizziness in the minocycline group	Minocycline safe and beneficial in RA
Tilley et al. 1995	219	Placebo	Randomized, double-blind, multicentre (median disease duration 8.5 years)	48 weeks	Significant improvement in clinical and lab parameters	Similar rates of toxicity in the two groups	Minocycline safe and effective for patients with mild to moderate RA
O'Dell et al. 1997	46	Placebo	Randomized double-blind (mean disease duration 4.5 months)	6 months	Significant improvement in number of 50% responders; no change in ESR	Similar rates of toxicity in the two groups; no discontinuations due to dizziness	Minocycline superior to placebo in early seropositive RA
O'Dell et al. 2001	60	Hydroxychloroquine (NB all patients also started on low-dose steroid)	Randomized, double-blline (mean disease duration 5.7 months)	2 years	Trend towards superior clinical and lab outcomes in minocycline group; significant superiority in terms of ACR 50 endpoint and requirement for steroid	Similar withdrawal rates in both groups; no withdrawals due to hyperpigmentation in minocycline group	Minocycline an effective DMARD in patients with early seropositive RA

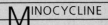

■ MINOCLYCLINE—GP INFORMATION SHEET

Recent studies have suggested that minocycline can act as a disease-modifying drug in RA. For this reason your patient has been started on minocycline.

Prescribing
The recommended initial dose is 50 mg bd continued for four weeks, increasing to 100 mg bd if tolerated.

Monitoring
FBC, urea and electrolytes, and liver function tests should be checked at baseline and then 3 monthly.

Adverse effects and management
The most commonly encountered side-effects are gastrointestinal upset and dizziness. Minocycline should be avoided in patients with vertigo. Minocyline can cause skin pigmentation after prolonged use (18 months or so).

Recent studies in the USA and Europe have reported cases of minocycline-induced lupus which can manifest as fever, skin rashes, mouth ulcers, photosensitivity, proteinuria and a positive ANA.

Management: Withdrawal of therapy. Most side-effects will reverse but skin changes persist for prolonged periods.

Patients on warfarin may require to have the dosage reduced while on minocycline. Iron preparations and antacids should not be taken within 3 hours of minocycline.

Possible toxicity
Female patients of child-bearing age are warned of the toxicity of this drug for the fetus during pregnancy and are therefore advised to take appropriate contraceptive measures.

3 DMARDs

A ZATHIOPRINE

INTRODUCTION

Azathioprine, a synthetic purine analogue, originated from attempts to alter the metabolism of 6-mercaptopurine. The similarity in appearance of immunoblastic lymphocytes to leukaemic cells prompted investigations of both drugs in modifying immune responses. When given at the time of sensitization it was possible to induce tolerance while retaining response to other antigens. Subsequent studies showed that azathioprine was superior to 6-mercaptopurine, in preventing rejection of canine renal allografts. Interest in its use in rheumatoid arthritis (RA) followed the observation that it was "beneficial, relatively safe and easy to manage", in recipients of allografts.

Although azathioprine is now seldom the disease-modifying antirheumatic drug (DMARD) of first choice, it remains a useful alternative when others have failed or if intercurrent illness make other DMARDs difficult to monitor in RA. It might therefore be chosen after use of sulphasalazine, methotrexate and gold or be used when proteinuria or azotaemia make these compounds less desirable.

PHARMACOLOGY

Azathioprine is virtually fully absorbed from the upper gastrointestinal tract. Peak plasma levels are achieved within 1–2 hours, little of the drug is protein bound and it is rapidly distributed. It does not cross the blood–brain barrier. Its action follows in vivo conversion to 6-mercaptopurine and within cells it is converted to purine thioanalogues. The key enzyme in the inactivation of thiopurines is thiopurine methyl transferase, which is inherited as an autosomal, co-dominant trait, with up to 12% of the population having low or negligible enzyme activity. Such individuals may be unusually sensitive to frequently used doses. There is some evidence that characterizing the phenotype may limit toxicity. In practice, access to this approach is limited.

■ BENEFIT

EVIDENCE OF BENEFIT

Table 1 shows studies comparing azathioprine with placebo
Table 2 shows clinical comparison with other DMARDs
Table 3 shows a meta-analysis
Table 4 shows radiological studies

Since much of the published work dates back 30 years, by current standards most is not acceptable. Table 1 shows the published placebo-controlled studies. In a meta-analysis of these, only three were of an appropriate standard or contained enough data to be included (see Table 2). The pooled data of 81 patients, of whom 40 received azathioprine, showed an improvement in joint count in favour of azathioprine. The change in erythrocyte sedimentation rate (ESR) also favoured azathioprine but it did not achieve statistical significance. There were insufficient data to make any comment on radiological or functional outcomes. Patients on azathioprine were five times more likely to withdraw than those on placebo, primarily owing to toxicity.

Comparative studies

These are shown in Table 1. In an 18-month study by Cade *et al.* (1976) azathioprine 2.5 mg/kg was compared with oral cyclophosphamide 1.5 mg/kg and intramuscular (IM) gold. Only 36 of the initial 121 patients completed 72 weeks of treatment. Toxicity leading to withdrwal was least with azathioprine (31% compared with 50% in the other groups), but cyclophosphamide was superior to both treatments when joint counts were compared. Erosion scores, function, and reduction in oral steroid were better in the patients on immunosuppressives.

In a study of radiological progression in 64 patients comparing 100–150 mg azathioprine daily to methotrexate 7.5–15 mg/week the number of new erosions was less in the methotrexate group, although the overall scores were not significantly different. The high number of dropouts in the azathioprine group may have been responsible. Methotrexate was clinically superior. Other studies have suggested a similar benefit in patients who receive azathioprine to penicillamine and methotrexate.

Azathioprine in other inflammatory arthritides

Most data come from case reports or small series of patients. There are data to support the use of azathioprine in psoriatic arthritis and there may be significant improvement in the skin.

In cases of overlap of RA with systemic lupus erythematosus (SLE), azathioprine may prove particularly useful.

Table 1 Azathioprine (AZA) in RA: placebo controlled

Reference	n	Comparative drugs	Study design/disease duration	Duration of follow-up (months)	Outcome efficacy	Outcome toxicity	Conclusion/ comment
Mason et al. 1969	49	Placebo AZA 2.5 mg/kg/day	Parallel Double-blind Seropositive erosive RA on 5 mg prednisolone for ≥ 6/12	52 weeks	Oral steroid use (4.3 mg down vs 0.75 mg in placebo)	5 withdrawals AZA. 9 with placebo. 2 macrocytic blood film, 2 leucopenia, 1 rash, 1 poor control	Drug with promise. Bone marrow suppression adequately monitored with monthly FBC. Need more information on long-term use and comparisons to other DMARDS
Woodland et al. 1981	28 (42)	AZA 2.5 mg/kg/day (n = 15) Placebo (n = 13)	Double-blind, parallel study Intention to treat Erosive disease of various duration	6 months	Pain score (change from baseline) SMD −1.05 (95% CI −1.85, −0.25) Morning stiffness, well-being, grip strength. No change in lab data	Withdrawals: 7/15 AZA 2.5, 4/14 AZA 1.25, 2/13 in placebo group. Most common side-effects included nausea and rash	Difficult to interpret results due to high drop-out rate. Dose of at least 2.5 mg required to obtain a significant improvement as judged by physicians blind to treatment

Study	N	Intervention	Design	Duration	Outcomes	Toxicity	Conclusions
Urowitz et al. 1973	19	AZA 2–2.5 mg/kg/day Placebo / 1 on concomitant Myocrisin	Crossover 13.6 year mean disease duration (SD 13.3) Analysis of completers	16 weeks × 2 (data at 16 weeks reported)	Swollen joints SMD −2.44 (95% CI −3.79, −1.10) (well-being, grip, active joint count, effusions, analgesia use, joint injection requirement, ESR, Ig, new erosions)	5 discontinued due to leucopenia	Statistic improvements in clinical variables but not for laboratory variables. Minimal toxicity where monitoring adequate. More long-term information needed
Hunter et al. 1975	17	AZA 2–2.5 mg/kg/day Placebo / 1 on concomitant Myocrisin	Double-blind, crossover at 16 weeks. Extended follow-up at 40 weeks. Active RA not responsive to gold or chloroquine therapy	40 months	Maintained initial response or further improvement	Nausea(1), leucopenia + thrombocytopenia(1). Increased chromosomal abnormalities	Sustained improvement in a difficult to treat patient group (12 of 17 remained on AZA at 40 months). Mild toxicity; but increased chromosomal abnormalities noted in AZA group only

Table 2 Azathioprine (AZA) in RA: Comparative studies (randomized monotherapy)

Reference	n	Comparative drugs	Study design/disease duration	Duration of follow-up (months)	Outcome efficacy	Outcome toxicity	Conclusion/comment
Halberg et al. 1984	74	AZA Levamisole Penicillamine	Double-blind Classical RA with active synovitis	48 months (2/3 withdrew prior to completion)	All drugs had similar efficacy—clinical and laboratory outcomes	Anaemia more common with AZA. Levamisole: unacceptable agranulocytosis	Similar benefit. Penicillamine felt to have fewer adverse effects
Hamdy et al. 1987	42	MTX low dose AZA	Controlled Classical RA, active synovitis not responsive to NSAID and conventional DMARDs	24 weeks	Both improved. No statistical difference; trend for faster improvement with MTX. Equivalent radiological progression	4 withdrew due to toxicity. 2 nausea (AZA/MTX) 1 rash (AZA) 1 LFT abnormal (MTX)	Similar benefit and toxicity
Currey et al. 1974	121	AZA 2.5 mg/kg/day Cyclophosphamide 1.5 mg/kg/day IM gold	Double-blind Active, seropositive erosive RA at diagnosis	18 months	Better joint counts with cyclophosphamide. Erosion scores function and lower steroid doses with cyclo/AZA better than gold	36 of 121 completed 72 weeks Least withdrawal from AZA group (31% vs 50%). Withdrawals due to GI, leucopenia or rash. None serious	Cyclophosphamide slightly more effective. AZA/cyclo had less radiological joint deterioration and more steroid-sparing effect. AZA had less short term toxicity

Study	n	Drugs	Design	Duration	Results	Toxicity	Conclusion
Berry et al. 1976	65	AZA, D-penicillamine	Single-blind, external observer	52 weeks	No significant difference	More AZA toxicity (10 vs 5). Nausea most common	Similar efficacy. More toxicity with AZA but not troublesome
Dwosh et al. 1977	33	AZA, Gold, Chloroquine	Early RA 11 per group less than 5 years' RA randomly assigned. Assessor blind to treatment 12, 24 weeks assessment clinical and laboratory measures	24 weeks	Equally effective. No placebo arm	Low toxicity	All equally effective. Azathioprine had greatest potential toxicity and could not be recommended over other DMARDs
Paulus et al. 1984	206	AZA 1.25–1.5 mg/kg/day, D-penicillamine 10–12 mg/kg/day (previous gold)	Double-blind controlled	24 weeks	No significant differences except lower ESR in penicillamine group. Improvement in most variables seen with both groups	LFT, leucopenia, GI upset	Similar benefit 134 completers
Jeurissen et al. 1991	64	AZA, MTX	Randomized, double-blind	48 weeks	Swollen joint count, pain score, ESR, CRP, HB, platelet, disease activity score	More AZA adverse effects	MTX faster more effective and less toxicity

Table 2 cont.

Reference	n	Comparative drugs	Study design/disease duration	Duration of follow-up (months)	Outcome efficacy	Outcome toxicity	Conclusion/ comment
Levy 1995	42	AZA Cyclophosphamide	Double-blind, controlled, crossover Abstract— inadequate information	6 months drug/6 months placebo	Statistical differences between drugs and placebo. Drug efficacy similar	Leucopenia and hypersensitivity with both (rarely)	Equally efficacious and reasonably well tolerated. Cyclophosphamide showed delayed hypersensitivity may make this less desirable in the long term
Willkens et al. 1995	209	AZA 50–150 mg/day MTX 5–15 mg/week AZA and MTX 5/50 7.5/100	RCT Probably not-intention-to-treat (110 patients on initial randomized regimen)	48 weeks	Clinical, laboratory, radiological. Responders defined as 30% improvement in 3 of 4 variables 38% combination, 26% AZA and 45% MTX (p=0.06). Trend towards reduced radiological progression with MTX	AZA and AZA + MTX more withdrawals due to toxicity	MTX alone is preferred treatment
Kruger 1992	117	AZA 1.5–2 mg/kg Cyclosporin A 5 mg/kg	Randomized double-blind multi-centre. Not intention-to-treat (92 completers)	6 months	Ritchie index, morning stiffness, grip strength, swollen joint count	9 adverse reaction, 1 loss of effect. Similar to cyclosporin	Efficacy and tolerability equal, but increased BP and creatinine seen only in cyclosporin group

Study	N	Drugs	Design	Duration	Efficacy	Withdrawal	Comments
Willkens et al. 1992	212	AZA MTX both	Randomized double-blind multi-centre Intention to treat (158 completers)	24 weeks	All >30% improvement AZA less effective than MTX/combination	GI side-effects and elevated liver enzymes most common reasons for withdrawal	MTX AZA + MTX more effective than AZA alone
Ahern et al. 1991	52	AZA (av 1.9 mg/kg) Cyclosporin A (mean 3.4 mg/kg)	Randomized double-blind	6 months	Both improved. No statistical difference	12 AZA withdrew. 6 GI, 4 loss of effect, 2 other. 7 cyclosporin withdrew	Similar. Careful monitoring required with cyclosporin to detect predictable side-effects
Arnold et al. 1990	53	AZA MTX	RCT	24 weeks, 3-year follow-up	No statistical difference	Similar dropout over 3 years. Similar rates of intolerance	Equivalent. Chance of treatment continuing beyond 18 months is low
Forre et al. 1987	24	AZA Cyclosporin	Open, controlled randomized study. No blinding	26 weeks	Cyclosporin significantly improved grip, Ritchie index, walking, PIP circumference global assessment by investigator. AZA grip only	Similar toxicity rates	Patients in cyclosporin group improved in more variables than AZA group

Table 3 Meta-analysis of studies of azathioprine (AZA) monotherapy in RA

Reference	n studies/patients	Therapies	Duration median	Outcome efficacy	Outcome toxicity	Verdict
Suarez-Almazor et al. 2002	40 AZA 41 placebo	AZA 2.0–3.0 mg/kg/day Placebo	6 months	Tender joint score SMD −0.98 (95% CI −1.45, −0.5) ESR difference not significant (−12.94) (Urowitz et al. 1973 only) Swollen joints SMD −2.44 (95% CI −3.79, −1.10) (Woodland et al. 1981 only) Pain score (change from baseline) SMD −1.05 (95% CI −1.85, −0.25)	4.6 times more likely to withdraw (CI 95% 1.16, 17.85) GI 15% [significant; OR 7.81 (95% CI 1.24, 49.19)] mucocutaneous 26% haematological 9%	Significant effect on disease activity. Small numbers from older trials. No assessment of long-term or functional outcome/radiological progression due to lack of data. Higher toxicity than other DMARDs. Not recommended over other DMARDs

Table 4 Radiological damage as outcome measure in RA azathioprine (AZA) studies

Reference	n	Comparative drugs	Study design	X-ray method	Outcome radiological scores	Conclusion
Jeurissen et al. 1991	64	AZA 100–150 mg MTX 7.5–15 mg weekly	Randomized, double-blind 48 weeks Intention-to-treat analysis	Modified Sharp score for hands. Feet also scored	11% and 43% of MTX and AZA respectively had progressed at 48 weeks	Less erosions in MTX group, but not significant. Trend for better clinical response in MTX group. Higher dropout from AZA group
Kerstens et al. 2000	64	AZA MTX	Open extension of randomized double-blind study 4 years Intention-to-treat	24 weeks, 48 weeks, 2 years and 4 years.	MTX significantly better than AZA at 2 years. Trend at 4 years (attributed to the fact that many of the original AZA patients were now treated with MTX)	MTX superior. More patients continued treatment with MTX

Combination therapy

In a descriptive study, 31 patients on a combination of immunosuppressives which included azathioprine identified from a cohort of 183 rheumatoid patients treated over a period of 10.5 years, 16 were in remission. The combination treatment duration ranged from 12 to 102 months and doses of immunosuppressives were low. Four of these patients developed malignancies during combination therapy, and three of them died.

In the efficacy studies referred to above, the main problems identified were upper gastrointestinal, marrow suppression (usually as leucopenia), hair thinning, zoster infection, rash and other hypersensitivity reactions.

■ HARM

Two principal sources exist for frequency of adverse events: the ACR guidelines for monitoring, and a sizeable post-marketing survey in the USA. The data are combined in Table 5.

Withdrawal of azathioprine follows an upper gastrointestinal problem in 60%; 10–15% stop therapy because of a haematologic problem and 5–10% following a rash. Other reasons for stopping azathioprine are rare, and whilst 3–7% stop because of an infection most will restart. In a prospective survey only two of 546 stopped azathioprine because of abnormal liver function tests.

In the same study the incidence of malignant tumours was 1.6% and "not significantly different from that observed in RA patients not taking any cytotoxic drug". In a 20-year follow-up study of rheumatoid patients given unusually high doses (up to 5 mg/kg) of azathioprine, the authors suggested an increased risk of lymphoma of one case per 1000 patient years of treatment. These results contrast with earlier reports in a variety of conditions treated with immunosuppression showing a 13.5 relative risk for reticuloendothelial cancer, most marked in post-transplant patients (58-fold.)

Dosage and monitoring

The ACR recommends 1–2 mg/kg body weight per day but doses up to 5 mg/kg have been used. Prior testing for the genotype of methylating enzymes is not widely practised and there may be added safety by introducing initial very low doses (e.g. 25 mg daily) and increasing the daily dose by a maximum of 25 mg initially every fortnight to a target if possible.

Drug interactions

The dose should be reduced by 75% in patients requiring concomitant allopurinol, and azathioprine should be avoided in patients taking ACE inhibitors if possible.

Hepatic and renal impairment

The dose should be reduced in patients with renal impairment. In the presence

Table 5 Adverse events during azathioprine (AZA) treatment

Adverse event	Dose related/idiosyncratic	Reversible	Occurs early or late	Frequency	What to do
Nausea/vomiting	Dose related	Yes	Early	About 10%	Antiemetics
Diarrhoea	?	Yes	Early	< 5%	Investigate and treat
Oral ulcers	?	Yes	?	< 5%	Check WBC
Rash/drug fever	Idiosyncratic	Yes	Early	< 5%	Stop AZA
Myelosuppression	Dose related	Yes	Early	< 5%	WBC <3/N<1.5 stop and re-introduce lower dose
Macrocytic anaemia	Dose related	Yes	Early	Common	Check B$_{12}$ folate monitor MCV and haemoglobin
Infections	Dose related	Yes	Any time	2% per annum	Treat Withhold AZA ?re-introduce
Abnormal LFTs	Idiosyncratic	Yes	Early	Rare	Stop AZA
Pancreatitis	Idiosyncratic	Usually	?	< 1%	Treat
Neoplasia, especially lymphoma	Idiosyncratic	If detected early	Late	In 4 of 31 who received AZA+HCQ+ cyclophosphamide OR 1 in 200 in patients on AZA >2 years	Stop AZA Suspect it

of elevated transaminases azathioprine treatment should be avoided unless started for autoimmune liver disease.

Monitoring

Monitoring is intended to minimize myelosuppression and complications such as sepsis, severe anaemia and bleeding. Before starting azathioprine checks of serum creatinine transaminases and full blood count (FBC) (including platelets and differential) are suggested. Checks of FBC are needed every 1–2 weeks during dosage increases and every four weeks in the long term.

In a survey of UK rheumatologists and an audit of three centres, the authors concluded that such intensive monitoring may be needed in the first six months but thereafter the frequency of haematological toxicity (133 patient years to observe one haematological adverse event in patients on azathioprine) monitoring is needed less often (at the time 75% of UK rheumatologists monitored FBC every four weeks.)

Compliance

Compliance may prove a problem with azathioprine, particularly when nausea is present. There may also be fear of complications of immunosuppressive therapy. If there is doubt about compliance, appropriate counselling should be given before proceeding to what appear to be unusually high doses.

Immunizations

Appropriate immunizations, such as flu vaccine, should be given, and there may be a case for other immunizations in patients with particular intercurrent health problems, such as respiratory disease, or patients known to have inadequate immunity to herpes zoster.

Contraindications
- Unexplained elevations of transaminases
- Previous intolerance of 6-mercaptopurine
- Concomitant enzyme inhibitor therapy (e.g. allopurinol, ACE inhibitors)—relative contraindication
- Known previous hypersensitivity reaction to azathioprine
- Planned conception
- Breast feeding

Family planning issues

Effects of azathioprine on fertility in both men and women have not been studied. In established pregnancy the rate of intrauterine growth retardation is up to 40%. Other risks include prematurity and temporary immunosuppression in the newborn. There remains the possibility of clinically important effects on the germline of the offspring. There are no data on azathioprine effects postpartum and in particular during breast feeding. The ACR considers that the hypothetical risk of immunosuppression in the infant outweighs the possible benefits.

■ SUMMARY

Azathioprine is likely to be used only after other agents of better proven benefits have been ruled out. Its main problem after establishing therapy is nausea. Clinically important myelosuppression can usually be avoided by gradual increases in dosage with fortnightly FBC checks. Care is needed to avoid drug interactions, especially with other drugs working through enzyme inhibition.

KEY REFERENCES

■ Urowitz *et al.* 1973

■ Woodland *et al.* 1981

■ Silman *et al.* 1988

■ Ahlmen *et al.* 1987

■ Black *et al.* 1998

■ AZATHIOPRINE—GP INFORMATION

Azathioprine is used to treat rheumatoid and similar inflammatory diseases. Toxicity can occur, but if precautions are taken most patients tolerate azathioprine without significant problems.

Delayed response is the norm, so patients need to continue their symptom-relieving therapy, although this can sometimes be reduced gradually, once a response to azathioprine occurs (usually 12–24 weeks).

Prescribing
Start at 25/50/75/100 mg per day
Increase the daily dose by 25 mg every 2/4 weeks to a target of __ mg/day

The final dose may be higher or lower, as the rate of metabolism of azathioprine varies widely from one person to another.

Contraindications
- Unexplained elevations of transaminases
- Previous intolerance of 6-mercaptopurine
- Concomitant enzyme inhibitor therapy (e.g. allopurinol, ACE inhibitors)—relative contraindication
- Known previous hypersensitivity reaction to azathioprine
- Planned conception
- Breast feeding

Drug interactions
- Suspect all enzyme inhibitors
- Reduce azathioprine dose by 75% if allopurinol started
- Contact the hospital if ACE inhibitors needed

Toxicity

nausea/vomiting	usually dose related, occurs in about 10%, try antiemetics
diarrhoea	occurs in <5%, try to treat it
oral ulcers	occurs in <5%, check WBC from FBC, consider oral swab for bacteriology
rash/drug fever	occurs **early** in <5%, stop azathioprine and seek other cause
myelosuppression	usually dose related and gradual, occurs in <5%; if WBC<3 OR neutrophils<1.5 stop azathioprine and reintroduce at lower dose
macrocytic anaemia	usually dose related, monitor
infections	usually dose related, occurs in about 2% per annum; treat promptly; annual flu vaccine
abnormal LFTs	idiosyncratic, rare; stop azathioprine
pancreatitis	idiosyncratic, <1%, stop azathioprine and treat
neoplasia	(especially lymphoma)—idiosyncratic, 1 in 200 on azathioprine >2 years, suspect it

Family planning

Women considering pregnancy should not take azathioprine.

The effect on children fathered by men on azathioprine is not known.

Contraception with IUCDs may be interfered with and alternative or additional contraceptive measures should be taken where appropriate.

Breast feeding is inadvisable where the mother is taking azathioprine.

Monitoring
We suggest:

FBC every 2 weeks whilst the dose is rising and then every 4 weeks for the first year of treatment (reducing frequency thereafter)

LFTs every 4 weeks till the dose is stable

Contact the hospital if:
WBC <4 and neutrophils <1.5 OR lymphocyte count <0.5
Platelets <120
Haemoglobin <9
AST/ALT consistently abnormal
Other difficulties arise

■ CHLORAMBUCIL—GP INFORMATION

Chlorambucil is used to treat refractory or complicated rheumatoid and similar inflammatory diseases. Toxicity can occur, but if precautions are taken most patients tolerate chlorambucil without significant problems.

Delayed response is the norm, so patients need to continue their symptom-relieving therapy, although this can sometimes be reduced gradually once a response to chlorambucil occurs (usually 12–24 weeks).

Prescribing
Start at 2 mg per day
Increase the daily dose by 2 mg every 2–4 weeks to a target dose of __ mg/day.

The final dose may be higher or lower as bone marrow sensitivity to chlorambucil varies widely from one person to another.

Contraindications
- Unexplained elevations of transaminases
- Known previous hypersensitivity reaction to chlorambucil
- Planned conception
- Breast feeding

Toxicity
- In >10%:
Rash
Myelosuppression (common and dose limiting)
- Onset 7 days
- Nadir 14 days
- Recovery 28 days (occasionally 6–8 weeks)
Abnormal liver enzymes—usually transient

- In 1–10%:
Hyperuricaemia
Menstrual cramps

cont.

■ In <1%:

Agitation, amenorrhoea, angioneurotic oedema, ataxia, chromosomal damage, confusion, fever, hallucinations, hepatic necrosis or other liver toxicity, infertility (may be irreversible), muscular twitching, myoclonic jerks, neoplasia especially acute myeloid leukaemia, neuropathy, seizures, tremor, weakness, interstitial pneumonitis or fibrosis, urticaria, infection.

NB: neoplasia (especially acute myeloid leukaemia)

Family planning

Known teratogenic effect, so men and women on chlorambucil should take appropriate contraceptive measures.

Breast feeding is contraindicated where the mother is taking chlorambucil.

Monitoring

We suggest:
FBC every 2 weeks whilst the dose is rising and then every 4 weeks for the first 6 months of treatment (reducing frequency thereafter).

LFTs every 4 weeks until the dose is stable.

Contact hospital if:

WBC < 4 × 10^9/L and neutrophils < 1.5 OR lymphocyte count < 0.5
Platelets < 120 × 10^9/L
Haemoglobin < 9 g/dL
AST/ALT consistently abnormal
Other difficulties arise

■ CHLORAMBUCIL—PATIENT INFORMATION SHEET

Chlorambucil helps control rheumatoid arthritis and its complications and similar conditions. It is also used in some other medical conditions.

How does chlorambucil work? Chlorambucil slows down the disease and damage caused by inflammation.

About two-thirds of patients will benefit from chlorambucil without ill effect, but you may not notice the improvement for 12 or more weeks. You will need to continue your usual treatment to keep symptoms under control, although you may be able to reduce this when the benefits of chlorambucil become apparent.

How do you take chlorambucil? You take it once or twice a day as tablets. The long-term dose is usually worked out according to your weight and is usually between 2 and 12 mg per day, but the starting dose is often low and the dose built up every 2 or 4 weeks. The dose may need to be adjusted according to side-effects or your response.

What are the side-effects? About one in 10 patients develop blood count problems and rash. Taking chlorambucil increases the risk of infections and you should tell your doctor if you become ill. Other problems that occur include nausea and period pains, and there are many rare side-effects.

Tell your doctor as soon as possible if you develop:
- Any unexplained bruising or bleeding
- Rash
- A high temperature or fever

Side-effects of chlorambucil usually develop gradually and go away gradually. Rarely malignancies, especially leukaemias, develop in patients taking chlorambucil.

Chlorambucil affects fertility and if you want to have children in the future you should discuss this when starting treatment—it may be possible to store eggs or sperm for future use.

Chlorambucil is only used in rheumatic diseases when the risks are outweighed by the potential benefits.

Blood tests You will need to have blood tests every 2 weeks to start with but once the dose has been stable for at least 4 weeks the tests can be reduced to every 4 weeks. Your family doctor can usually perform these.

You will be given a monitoring card to carry and the results will be written on this. Please make sure the card is up to date when you bring it to the clinic.

Pregnancy You should not start chlorambucil if you are planning a family in the foreseeable future. It would probably harm the unborn child.

It also should not be taken when breast feeding.

Men on chlorambucil should not father children, as it would probably harm the unborn child.

Other medicines and alcohol If you need other medicines tell your doctor and the pharmacist you are taking chlorambucil.

As chlorambucil sometimes (rarely) affects the liver it is wise to drink as little alcohol as possible during the first 3 months of treatment. After this it is safe to drink alcohol with this drug but too much is always dangerous.

3 DMARDs

CYCLOSPORIN

> **KEY INDICATIONS**
> - Rheumatoid arthritis
> - Psoriatic arthritis
> - Systemic lupus erythematosus

INTRODUCTION

The successful use of cyclosporin in the prevention of immune-mediated solid organ transplantation rejection led to initial open-label studies in rheumatoid arthritis (RA) as early as 1979. Subsequently, double-blinded randomized placebo-controlled trials have confirmed the efficacy of cyclosporin in RA and it is currently used to treat a wide spectrum of rheumatolgical disorders, including psoriatic arthritis and systemic lupus erythematosus.

However, RA remains the only arthropathy that is a licensed indication for treatment with cyclosporin in the United Kingdom, and the evidence base for the use of use of cyclosporin in RA is far stronger than for other rheumatological conditions. In the treatment of RA, cyclosporin is considered a second or third choice of disease-modifying antirheumatic drug (DMARD) either alone or in combination with methotrexate.

PHARMACOLOGY

Cyclosporin effect and toxicity is dose dependent. Cyclosporin is metabolized by the cytochrome P450 isoenzyme CYP 3A4. Drugs may alter cyclosporin levels by inducing or inhibiting this enzyme. Cyclosporin is also transported back into the gut lumen by the intestinal P (multi-drug resistant) glycoprotein, which is also inducible and inhibitable by other drugs.

BENEFIT

The one-year efficacy of cyclosporin in the treatment of severe, active refractory RA has been established in three placebo-controlled randomized controlled trials (Tugwell *et al.* 1990; Dougados *et al.* 1988; Forre 1994), and confirmed by meta-

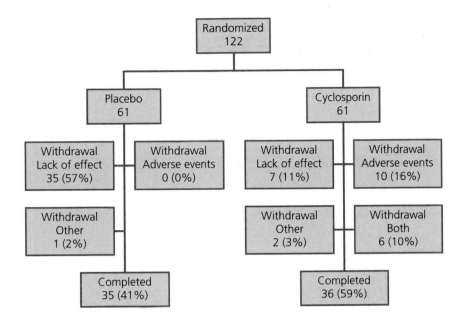

Figure 1 Oystein Forre and the Norwegian Arthritis Study Group. *Arthritis Rheum* 1994; **37**: 1506–1512.

analysis (Wells *et al.* 2000). The Forre trial (1994) compared cyclosporin with placebo and provides typical results with improvements in disease activity, physical function and radiological progression, as shown in Tables 1 and 2. Meta-analysis of the three studies confirms significant improvements in clinical joint scores and function, but the changes in acute phase reactants were not significant.

■ PROSPECTIVE DOUBLE-BLIND RANDOMIZED CONTROLLED TRIALS

Cyclosporin has equal efficacy to intramuscular (IM) gold, azathioprine, D-penicillamine and mthotrexate. In an open-label study, cyclosporin treatment in early RA resulted in a statistically significant reduction in radiological joint damage of patients when compared to patients taking either auranofin, hydroxychloroquine, IM gold or penicillamine.

These findings are summarized in Table 3.

■ COMBINATION TREATMENT

In a randomized, double-blind controlled trial, cyclosporin plus methotrexate was superior to methotrexate alone in RA patients selected because of a partial

Table 1 Change in outcome measures at 48 weeks (cyclosporin vs placebo)

Mean value ± standard error of mean

	Cyclosporin (n = 61)	Placebo (n = 61)	p Value
Ritchie Articular Index (max. 87)	–7.7 ± 1.6	–2.4 ± 1.4	<0.01
No. of swollen joints (max. 22)	–3.6 ± 0.6	–0.3 ± 0.5	<0.001
Overall assessment of treatment			
Patient (max. 4)	2.02 ± 0.2	0.79 ± 0.16	<0.001
Physician (max. 4)	1.79 ± 0.19	0.67 ± 0.14	<0.001
Erythrocyte sedimentation rate	–3.5 ± 4.7	–2.0 ± 3.9	NS
C-reactive protein	–13.4 ± 8.0	+5.0 ± 15.8	NS
Lee Functional Index (max. 36)	–2.2 ± 0.7	1.8 ± 0.7	<0.001

No data available on ACR remission rates in three randomized controlled trials of cyclosporin.

Table 2 Reduction in radiographic progression (cyclosporin vs placebo)

Mean value ± standard error of mean

	Cyclosporin (n = 37)	Placebo (n = 23)
Baseline Larsen score	1.61 ± 0.16	1.43 ± 0.11
Increase in Larsen score (48 weeks)	–0.01 ± 0.04*	0.17 ± (0.05)
Baseline no. of erosions	5.16 ± 0.73	4.14 ± 0.61
Change in no. of erosions (48 weeks)	0.06 ± 0.00**	1.03 ± 0.35

*$p < 0.004$ cyclosporin vs placebo; **$p < 0.04$ cyclosporin vs placebo.

response to methotrexate (Tugwell *et al.* 1995). However, intensive treatment of early RA with a poor prognosis by methotrexate, cyclosporin and intra-articular corticosteroids was not superior to monotherapy with sulphasalazine at 48 weeks of follow-up (Proudman *et al.* 2000). Similarly, while the treatment of early RA with methotrexate and cyclosporin produced a clinical response at six months,

Table 3 Results from double-blind randomized controlled trials comparing cyclosporin with other DMARDs

Comparator drug	Comparison with cyclosporin	Study population
IM gold (Kvien et al. 2002)	Equal efficacy	Early disease
Methotrexate (Drosos et al. 2000)*	Equal efficacy	Early disease
Azathioprine (Kruger et al. 1994)	Equal efficacy	Established disease
Penicillamine	Equal efficacy	Established disease
Auranofin **Hydroxychloroquine** **Leflunomide** **Sulphasalazine** **Etanercept** **Infliximab**	No data	

*Not double-blinded.

cyclosporin was inferior to methotrexate as continuation "step-down" monotherapy (Marchesoni et al. 2002)

■ TOXICITY

Up to 15% of RA patients treated with cyclosporin require withdrawal of therapy within the first year of treatment, owing to an adverse event (Table 4). In a meta-analysis of three trials comparing cyclosporin and placebo for up to one year, the commonest side-effects of cyclosporin were headache, tremor, nausea, dyspepsia, gum hyperplasia and parasthesia. Renal toxicity and hypertension is dose related and predictable with careful monitoring of patients during dose escalation or introduction of other medications. Long-term high-dose (>5 mg/kg/day) cyclosporin is associated with irreversible progressive renal damage. The risk of this is very low in RA patients managed according to current guidelines (≤ 5 mg/kg/day).

Serious and life-threatening toxicity is uncommon. Opportunistic infection occurs rarely, and patients with a history of herpes simplex or zoster infection should be advised to present for treatment early. Malignancy may occur in patients taking cyclosporin in the long term. A review of 1000 patients with RA found 17 cases of cancer; this was not increased when compared with the risk of malignancy of other DMARDs. The combination of methotrexate and cyclosporin does not appear to increase serious side-effects significantly. There are very few long-term toxicity studies of cyclosporin.

Table 4 Cyclosporin adverse events

Adverse event	Frequency	Timescale and nature	Recommended action
Cardiovascular Hypertension Oedema	Common	Dose related	If BP rises to abnormal range for age, consider 25–50% dose reduction or cessation of cyclosporin. Consider renal cause of oedema
Renal Nephropathy	Common	Dose-related effect on GFR is reversible. Long-term high-dose associated with irreversible renal damage	Consider 25–50% dose reduction or cessation of cyclosporin. Risk is increased in the elderly. Avoid other nephrotoxic drugs including NSAIDs and radiocontrast agents where possible
CNS/PNS Headaches Tremor	Common	Dose related	Rule out other causes. Consider 25–50% dose reduction or cessation of cyclosporin
Dermatological Hirsutism Hypertrichosis	Common	Occurs to a degree in 4–8 weeks in all patients	A severe degree of hypertrichosis may necessitate discontinuation. Resolution takes several months
Infections	Common	Any time; increase in herpes simplex and zoster may occur; other opportunistic infections reported, but rare	Continue treatment during minor infection; suspend therapy in severe or opportunistic infection

Gastrointestinal Nausea/vomiting Diarrhoea Gum hyperplasia Dyspepsia	Common	Oral antiemetics and antidiarrhoea medication may be effective; try dose reduction. Severe gum hyperplasia may necessitate discontinuation, and Resolution takes several months
Malignancy	Rare	Mechanism may be due to long-term cumulative effect of immunosuppression	Lymphoma and skin neoplasia. Risk of malignancy on cyclosporin is similar to that of other DMARDs
Haematological Leucopenia Anaemia	Rare	Idiosyncratic	Suspend or reduce therapy if there is any sudden unexplained drop in WCC or haemoglobin
Hepatic	Very rare	Idiosyncratic	Hyperbilirubinaemia. Severe hepatotoxicity is a feature of overdosage

■ MONITORING

The British Society of Rheumatology (BSR) has produced guidelines for the monitoring of cyclosporin therapy in the treatment of RA (see Table 5).

Patients should be given oral and written information about cyclosporin therapy, and the potential for side-effects. Patients should be advised to seek medical help in the event of unexplained fever, sore throat, bleeding, bruising, rash or jaundice.

■ DRUG INTERACTIONS (see Table 6)

- There are numerous drug interactions involving cyclosporin. It is recommended that the data sheet be consulted at the time of first prescription and if any other drugs are introduced.
- In particular, the dose of diclofenac should be halved if cyclosporin is co-prescribed.
- Colchicine should be avoided.
- Potassium-sparing diurectics should be used with caution.
- Grapefruit juice should be avoided.

Monitoring of cyclosporin blood levels is not essential but may be useful in detecting drug interactions or noncompliance.

■ PRACTICAL PRESCRIBING (see Table 7)

The co-prescription of other nephrotoxic agents should be avoided where practically possible. When possible, reduce NSAID dosage by substituting with simple or compound analgesics. There is no evidence that cycloxygenase–2-selective inhibitors are less nephrotoxic than nonselective NSAIDs when used in combination with cyclosporin.

Cyclosporin has proved to be an effective and relatively well-tolerated drug, but dose-related renal toxicity and hypertension limit the therapeutic dose and necessitate careful monitoring of renal function and blood pressure. Relatively few patients with RA have remission induced by cyclosporin therapy. Subsequently, cyclosporin may be used in combination with methotrexate. The addition of cyclosporin to parenteral gold did not have a superior efficacy to placebo in combination with parenteral gold. The efficacy of cyclosporin in combination with other DMARDs remains to be determined.

Table 5 BSR guidelines for monitoring cyclosporin therapy

Blood pressure	Baseline (at least twice). Every fortnight until dose stable for 3 months. Monthly thereafter	If BP rises to abnormal range for age, consider 25–50% dose reduction or cession of cyclosporin
Urea and creatinine	Baseline. Every fortnight until dose stable for 3 months. Monthly thereafter	If creatinine rises >30% above baseline, repeat creatinine estimation and consider 25–50% dose reduction or cessation of cyclosporin. Avoid cyclosporin in moderate/severe renal impairment
Full blood count	Baseline. Monthly until dose is stable. 3-monthly thereafter*	Withold cyclosporin if unexplained bruising or platelets <150×10⁹/L
AST/ALT	Baseline. Monthly until dose is stable. 3-monthly thereafter*	Stop or reduce dose by 25–50% if unexplained >2-fold increase in transaminases
Lipids	Baseline. 6-monthly thereafter	If significant rise in lipids consider 25–50% dose reduction. Cyclosporin increases levels of lovastatin, atorvastatin and simvastatin and may increase the risk of rhabdomyloysis

*Perform monthly if used in combination with methotrexate.

Table 6 Drug interactions		
Nephrotoxic agents	NSAIDs, radiocontrast agents	Avoid or reduce dose when practically possible. Consider non-nephrotoxic alternatives
↓**Cyclosporin levels**	***Antiepileptics:*** phenytoin,* carbamazepine,* primidone ***Antibiotics:*** rifampicin,* sulphonamides, trimethoprim	*These agents may double the rate of elimination of cyclosporin
↑**Cyclosporin levels**	***Antibiotics:*** erythromycin, clarithromycin, fluoroquinolones ***Antifungals:*** ketaconazole, itraconazole, fluconazole ***Calcium channel blockers:*** Diltiazem, verapamil, nicardipine, amlodipine ***Other:*** colchicine, amiodarone, H$_2$ blockers, grapefruit juice	
Effect of cyclosporin on drug metabolism	***HMG CoA reductase inhibitors:*** simvastatin, lovastatin, atorvastatin Digoxin	May increase levels and risk of rhabdomyolysis. Does not interact with pravastatin and fluvastatin Increase levels of digoxin
Vaccination	Avoid live vaccines	Annual flu vaccine is recommended

Table 7 Practical prescribing of cyclosporin in RA

Dose		
Initial dose:	2.5 mg/kg/day	Take in 2 equal divided doses. Increase dose at 8 weeks if insufficient response. Increase again at 12 weeks if insufficient response. Discontinue if insufficient response after 12 weeks on maximal tolerated dose. Consider co-prescription of methotrexate if partial response
Increments:	0.5–0.75 mg/kg/day	
Maximum dose:	4 mg/kg/day	
Preparation	Microemulsion (Neoral)	Increase absorption and reduced variability. The bioavailability of Sandimmun and Neoral is not equal, and careful monitoring is advised if changing preparations
Contraindications	Uncontrolled hypertension Renal impairment Past or current malignancy Hypersensitivity to cyclosporin	
Cautions	Elderly Multiple drug interactions Nephrotoxic drugs Dose-related nephrotoxicity	Renal impairment is more frequent in elderly patients. Use caution with other potentially nephrotoxic drugs
Alcohol	Advise moderation	No specific interaction with cyclosporin
Pregnancy	Contraindicated	Cyclosporin crosses the placenta and use during pregnancy is associated with premature birth and low birth weight
Breast feeding	Contraindicated	Cyclosporin is secreted in breast milk

SUMMARY

- Cyclosporin is a suitable "second choice" DMARD in patients with active RA who have not responded to other DMARDs.
- Cyclosporin improves disease activity and physical function, and reduces radiological progression.
- Serious toxicity is uncommon and dose related. Monitoring of renal function and blood pressure is required to minimize risk.
- Although effective and relatively well tolerated, drug dose-related renal toxicity and hypertension limit its therapeutic potential.
- Relatively few patients with RA have remission induced by cyclosporin alone.
- It may be used in combination with methotrexate.
- The efficacy of cyclosporin in combination with other DMARDs remains to be determined.

KEY REFERENCES

- Tugwell *et al.* 1990

- Dougados *et al.* 1998

- Forre 1994

- Wells *et al.* 2000

- Tugwell *et al.* 1995

■O ral cyclophosphamide

This is not a wine for drinking. This is a wine for laying down and avoiding.

(Monty Python)

KEY INDICATIONS

- Rheumatoid arthritis
- Systemic lupus erythematosus
- Vasculitis
- Wegener's granulomatosis
- Rarities

■ INTRODUCTION

Cyclophosphamide (CP) is an alkylating agent which crosslinks DNA so that it cannot replicate. Its main effect is on rapidly dividing cells. It is toxic to dividing and resting T- and B-cells, and reduces the number of active T- and B-cells.

Oral absorption is excellent (>90% bioavailability) so in this respect there is little advantage to intravenous therapy. CP itself is inactive and is metabolized in the liver. Phosphoramide mustard is the principal active metabolite. Acrolein, excreted in the urine, is thought to be responsible for most of the urothelial toxicity. Excretion is predominantly renal, so renal impairment demands dose reduction.

When few alternative disease-modifying antirheumatic drugs (DMARDs) existed there was interest in CP to control articular inflammation in rheumatoid arthritis (RA). As the number of DMARDs has expanded CP has become almost redundant for arthritis, but retains a valuable role in the treatment of extra-articular disease (e.g. vasculitis and neuropathy). Its principal current rheumatological use is in vasculitis, lupus and Wegener's granulomatosis. The reason for the now rare use of CP for arthritis is simple—toxicity.

There is no better illustration of the therapeutic tightrope a rheumatologist will ask his patients to tread. The use of CP exemplifies crucial practice points important for all DMARDs:

- Communication with the patient to appreciate therapeutic goals and toxicity
- Good local liaison with general practitioners about monitoring
- Good communication to ensure that toxicity is addressed promptly and early

More than with any other DMARD there is constant dose adjustment (usually reduction) according to toxicity, vigilance for early signs of toxicity and continued attention long after the drug has been withdrawn.

■ EFFICACY OF ORAL CP

Support for the use of CP comes from small studies performed long ago. A Cochrane systematic review in 2002 (Suarez-Almazor et al. 2002) identified just two placebo-controlled trials of acceptable quality, the total number of patients receiving CP being 31. These two studies were: Cooperating Clinics Committee (CCC) of the ARA (n = 20 on CP up to 150 mg/day, median dose about 100 mg/day for 32 weeks) published in 1970, and Townes et al. (n = 11, CP mean 1.8 mg/kg/day vs placebo for 9 months) reported in 1976.

It is salutary to note that for a confident calculation to detect a 40% difference between groups and avoid a type II error, each limb of a CP study would need 200 patients.

The CCC study showed that 15 of 20 patients (75%) improved in at least four of five disease activity measures after 32 weeks compared with seven of 28 (25%) of the comparator group (on 15 mg/day CP, considered a placebo). There was dramatic reduction of early morning stiffness, number of painful joints and number of swollen joints between baseline and study end. A nonsignificant modest fall in erythrocyte sedimentation rate (ESR) was observed.

In the first limb of a crossover study, Townes et al. (1976) showed substantial and statistically significant improvement in number of painful joints (11 of 11 improved), number of swollen joints (11 of 11 improved) and EMS. Again there was a trend (seven of 11 improved) but not statistically significant for a fall in ESR. Eight of 11 CP-treated subjects showed improvement in all five measures compared to just one of 11 in the placebo group.

Calculation of ACR response rates and number needed to treat is not possible from the data available in these mostly three-decade-old studies.

The effective dose of CP has received attention: 15 mg was assumed to be equivalent to placebo (CCC) and 0.87–1 mg/kg/day in a small study (Lidsky 1973) was no better than placebo; 50 mg/day (Keysser et al. 1998, dose in mg/kg not stated or calculable) was inadequate—48% had withdrawn for inefficacy by one year. The CCC found benefit from a median daily dose of approximately 100 mg—the precise dose and dose/kg cannot be calculated from the report. Williams et al. (1980) showed similar efficacy with target doses of 75 or 150 mg/day (n = 44 each limb; mean dose and dose/kg not stated and not calculable). Smyth et al. (1975) found prednisolone plus CP 75 mg (n = 13, 1.1 mg/kg mean) substantially better than prednisolone plus placebo. A separate open study of 105 mg/day (1.7 mg/kg/day) by Smyth et al. also reported substantial and significant improvement in various measures in 19 patients. The effective dose is probably at least 75–100 mg per day.

Currey et al. (1974) compared CP (1.5 mg/kg/day, n = 39), Myocrisin[®]

(n = 38) and azathioprine (2.5 mg/kg/day, n = 44) for 18 months. CP was considered slightly the more effective drug with a 65% improvement in the functional capacity score, and a 66% mean reduction of the initial score for number of joints involved.

Clinical effect is usually seen by two months and is maximal by around five to seven months. Relapse begins within two months of cessation.

■ DOES CP AFFECT X-RAY PROGRESSION?

It seems likely that there is a reduction in radiological progression with CP. We cannot be sure given the relatively unsophisticated scoring systems employed and the manner of reporting.

Currey et al. (1974) reported that CP was better than intramuscular (IM) gold at retarding X-ray progression, with no placebo group. The CCC (1970) showed more bone destruction in the "placebo" group—half the "placebo" group developed new or worsened erosions compared to 10% of the high dose CP group. Townes et al. (1976) found the mean number of new erosions to be 1.9 in the CP group and 4.3 in the placebo group. They attributed the benefit of CP to "extreme progression in two patients" on placebo and seemed to have an unreliable scoring system.

■ TOXICITY

Cyclophosphamide toxicity seriously limits its use (see Table 1). Toxicity tends to be dose dependent.

Long-term follow-up studies of CP-treated patients show that malignancy may develop many years after CP has been discontinued. The cumulative incidence of malignancy increases with time.

CP is frequently toxic, often seriously so, and death due to neutropenic sepsis has been reported. Long-term cumulative oncogenicity leaves a worrying legacy long after the drug may have been discontinued.

Urothelium
Urothelial toxicity is the major worry. Complications include dysuria without haemorrhage (9–45%), haemorrhagic cystitis (10–43%), asymptomatic microscopic haematuria (up to 45%), bladder fibrosis and bladder cancer. It seems likely that cystitis and fibrosis are linked to an increased risk of bladder cancer.

Malignancy
Malignancy following treatment of RA with CP 50 mg to 150 mg daily was studied by Baker et al. (1987). The relative risk of any malignancy was 2.3 for the CP-treated group compared with similar but non-CP-treated controls. The increased risk was obvious from six years after the first CP dose and persisted for

Table 1 Cyclophosphamide toxicity

Adverse event	Frequency	Timescale and nature	Action/comment
Haemorrhagic cystitis	10–43%	During or even long after use. Dose related	Stop CP. Check Hb. Cystoscopy. Long-term surveillance for bladder cancer. Do not restart CP
Dysuria without blood	20–45%	During use	Increase oral fluids
Microscopic haematuria	Up to 45%	During/after use	Cystoscopy
Alopecia	Up to 63%	Dose dependent	Reduce dose if severe
Herpes zoster	5% by 9 months		Antiviral treatment (may need IV)
Other infections	Up to 24%	During use	Stop CP until resolved. If infection severe, no more CP
Amenorrhoea	Common	During use	May induce menopause
Infertility	Common	During/after use	Usually irreversible. ?store gametes
Teratogenicity	Very common	During and ? after	Immaculate contraception
Nausea/vomiting	20–64%	During use	Oral antiemetics or dose reduction
Stomatitis	0–29%	During use	Dose reduction
Leucopenia	Common	Highly dose dependent	If WBC < 3.5—reduce dose 50% If WBC < 2.5—stop CP until >3.5

at least 13 years. The main risk factors identified were mean total CP dose, duration of use and tobacco use, of which the most important was total CP dose. Four of six patients (66%) developing bladder cancer had preceding haemorrhagic cystitis.

Only slightly reassuring was the finding that mortality from malignancy was identical in men treated with CP vs men not treated with CP (although it was greater amongst women treated with CP than in those not treated with CP). This is partly because the most numerous malignancies were those of the skin and bladder. There are implications for prolonged surveillance after CP cessation.

Talar-Williams et al. (1996) reported on 145 patients treated with oral CP for Wegener's granulomatosis with a median follow-up of 8.5 years (range 0.5–27 years). Their estimated incidence of bladder carcinoma since first CP dose was 2% at 5 years, 5% at 10 years and 16% at 15 years. They stressed that these figures were likely to be underestimates. This represented a 31-fold increased incidence of bladder carcinoma compared to the general population of the USA.

Patients took CP 2 mg/kg/day for at least one year after complete remission of symptoms, then 25 mg decrements every two to three months, as possible. CP dose was adjusted to keep absolute neutrophil count greater than 1.0×10^9/L. Smoking greatly increased the risk of transitional cell bladder carcinoma. The latency period for detection of malignancy ranged from seven months to 15 years. New tumours were still being detected up to 10 years after cessation of therapy.

Nonglomerular microscopic haematuria was the only variable associated with bladder cancer. Routine urinalysis for nonglomerular haematuria was recommended every three to six months ad infinitum, and cystoscopy in those with haematuria. Urine cytology was not useful for monitoring for development of bladder cancer.

Haemorrhagic cystitis

Haemorrhagic cystitis may be minor or very severe. Bleeding may continue for up to three months, necessitating multiple transfusions. A substantial proportion of these patients develop bladder cancer. Of the 119 patients of Baker et al. (1987), 16 had haemorrhagic cystitis, four (25%) of whom developed bladder cancer. Early reports from the CCC (1970) suggested that CP could be restarted after this complication—with present knowledge, permanent withdrawal of CP is wiser.

Dysuria

Dysuria without haemorrhage occurs in 20–45% of patients. It is not clear from reports whether these patients subsequently develop haemorrhagic cystitis or bladder fibrosis.

It is not established whether concomitant daily oral treatment with mesna abolishes the excess urothelial toxicity of chronic low-dose oral CP.

Haematological

Care must be taken when examining a white blood cell count (WBC) report not to miss a marked lymphopenia hidden within an acceptable total white cell population.

Known marrow-suppressive effects of CP demand constant attention to full blood count (FBC) monitoring, especially for neutrophils and to some extent lymphocytes. Most trial regimes have aimed to keep the total WBC count above 3500 or the neutrophil count above 1000. Especially after a year of treatment, cumulative marrow sensitivity often means that ever smaller doses are needed to maintain an acceptable WBC count.

Of those receiving 150 mg/day of CP, 32% had a WBC count less than 3500 compared to 6% receiving 75 mg/day. Only 4% of patients withdrew because of leucopenia in that study, compared to 35% withdrawing for leucopenia in the study of the CCC. Reassuringly, a WBC count between 1.5 and 2.5×10^9/L returned to above 3.5×10^9/L within one week in half of the affected patients and in all by three weeks of either dose reduction or discontinuation.

Thrombocytopenia is rare. A minor fall in haemoglobin in some studies is difficult to interpret.

Baker *et al.* (1987) found five malignancies in 119 rheumatoid patients treated with CP—two non-Hodgkin's lymphomas, two acute leukaemias and one myeloma—a substantial increase compared with the control group (see Table 2).

Infection

Within nine months of starting CP, 5% of patients develop herpes zoster. Studies have not told us whether these patients had leuco/lymphopenia. Urinary tract infections are reported in up to 68% of study patients. Serious sepsis, sometimes fatal, is frequently reported. Gaffney and Scott (1998) reported severe bacterial infections in "only 12% of patients receiving pulse CP for a variety of indications". Often there is the compounding effect of co-prescribed corticosteroids.

Alopecia

This is common and of variable severity. Severe (by subjective definition) alopecia is reported in 16–35% on oral CP with up to 63% of patients reporting some degree of alopecia. Frequency and severity are dose related (Williams *et al.* 1980). In 1975, Smyth *et al.* offered the following good news: "Alopecia was common, but in this era, when wearing a wig is popular, this complication was accepted with little objection."

Reproductive system

Oral CP may induce the menopause. In the CCC trial (1970) (median dose approximately 100 mg/day) all three premenopausal women at inception who completed six months of treatment developed amenorrhoea. At a mean daily dose of 105 mg or 1.7 mg/kg for only six months, three patients developed amenorrhoea persisting for at least four years (Smyth *et al.* 1975).

Irreversible infertility or decreased fertility occur in men and women. The

Table 2 Malignancy associated with cyclophosphamide

Adverse event	Frequency	Timescale and nature	Action
Bladder cancer	2% after 5 years 5% after 10 years 16% after 16 years	Dose dependent. More common in smokers	Vigilance and early referral. Routine urinalysis may detect early cancer

Other malignancy
  Skin cancer
  blood/lymphoreticular
	Overall
	relative
	risk = 2.3
		Indefinite risk.
		Probably increases
		with time
			Vigilance and early
			referral

incidence in RA is not known. Azoospermia, amenorrhoea and induced menopause are more likely with increasing age at treatment, higher CP dose and longer duration of treatment. Currey *et al.* (1974), (1.5 mg/kg/day) found it worrying that all six men on CP who were tested had azoospermia.

CP is teratogenic. Effective contraception is mandatory for women receiving this drug. Pregnancy should be excluded before starting CP in women of childbearing potential.

Gastrointestinal
Nausea and vomiting are common. The low frequency of withdrawal for this reason from drug studies is in contrast to the author's own experience. In one study recorded as "minimal, never lasting or troublesome" 20–64% of the patients experienced nausea and 8–45% experienced vomiting (Townes *et al.* 1976). Diarrhoea is occasionally reported.

Stomatitis is reported in 0–29% of study patients.

Other CP-attributable adverse events
There may be a 10–20% reduction in immunoglobulin levels, which return to normal on drug discontinuation. There is a marked inhibition of response to primary immunization during CP treatment, but seemingly no effect on primary humoral immune response or delayed skin response to tuberculin or mumps antigen (see Tables 3 and 4).

Table 3 Systems unaffected by chronic oral cyclophosphamide

- Liver rarely affected
- No neurotoxicity
- Blood pressure unaffected
- Pneumonitis rarely if ever
- Significant drug interactions are rare

These modest consolations are not usually adequate to outweigh the numerous disadvantages.

Table 4 Contraindications to use of cyclophosphamide for RA

Absolute contraindications
Current or planned pregnancy
Breast feeding
Previous urothelial malignancy
Previous severe reaction to CP—including previous haemorrhagic cystitis
Active infection, especially tuberculosis

Relative contraindications
Low WBC count
Bronchiectasis or recurrent infections
Previous malignancy
Renal impairment (adjust dose)

■ USE AND MONITORING

- Cyclophosphamide is available in the UK as 50 mg tablets.
- The British Society for Rheumatology has not produced guidelines for monitoring CP.

In the UK the Arthritis Research Campaign publishes a patient information leaflet on CP, available on the Internet: www.arc.org.uk.

Record details of discussion and warnings in the patients' notes.

Women of child-bearing potential must have pregnancy excluded before treatment and they must practise effective contraception. Breast feeding is not permitted.

- Patients should be given oral and written information about CP therapy and the potential side-effects, including the long-term risks. Advise smokers to stop. Patients should be advised to seek medical help in the event of unexplained fever, sore throat, bleeding or bruising. All infections must be treated promptly and WBC checked urgently.
- A high fluid intake is recommended to minimize urothelial exposure to acrolein. For patients with reduced mobility due to pain or joint damage this may be a recommendation difficult to follow, owing to the practical difficulties of frequent visits to the toilet.
- Start CP 50 mg/day with weekly FBC. After one month if tolerated increase to 100 mg/day. If tolerated, aim for a maximum of either 150 mg/day or 2 mg/kg/day after two months. If WBC stable for a further month, check WBC every two weeks.
- If WBC between 3.5 and 2.5×10^9/L reduce dose by 50%.
- If WBC $< 2.5 \times 10^9$/L stop CP until WBC $> 3.5 \times 10^9$/L then re-introduce at 50% of preceding dose.
- If neutrophils $<1.5 \times 10^9$/L, stop CP until $>2.0 \times 10^9$/L, then re-introduce at 50% of preceding dose.
- Dipstix urinalysis for haematuria at time of each blood test.
- Offer annual flu vaccination. Avoid live vaccines. Although unsupported by evidence it seems prudent to offer pneumococcal vaccine, preferably before starting CP.
- Warn patients that if they have not had chicken-pox but come into contact with someone who has chicken-pox or shingles, or if the patient develops either chicken-pox or shingles they should seek medical attention immediately to prevent disseminated viral disease.
- Monitoring for lymphoproliferative and other malignant disease seems appropriate but undefined. Once off CP, regular urinalysis for haematuria may help early detection of bladder cancer.

SUMMARY FOR RA INFLAMMATORY JOINT DISEASE

- CP is rarely suitable for active inflammatory joint disease in RA
- Only to be initiated by experienced rheumatologists
- Meticulous monitoring during use is mandatory
- Serious toxicity almost precludes CP use for those still wishing to have children
- Serious increased risk of malignancy makes long-term supervision essential

KEY REFERENCES

■ Baker *et al.* 1987

■ Cooperating Clinics Committee 1970

■ Suarez-Almazor *et al.* 2002

■ Talar-Williams *et al.* 1996

■ Townes *et al.* 1976

3 DMARDs

Cytokine-targeting therapies

■ INTRODUCTION

The precise aetiology of most inflammatory arthropathies remains unclear. Recent studies have clearly defined the presence and functional importance of pro-inflammatory cytokines in the perpetuation of synovial inflammation.

■ Cytokines are peptides that exist in families of related molecules. They function by binding to a specific receptor on a target cell and thereby facilitate communication within the immune system between cells that may be required to operate in a co-ordinated manner but which may be situated some distance apart. Specifically, studies in rodent arthritis models and in human inflammatory synovial membrane models have established the predominance of pro-inflammatory vs anti-inflammatory cytokines in driving articular inflammation. Tumour necrosis factor (TNFα) and interleukin-1 (IL-1) represent prototypic pro-inflammatory cytokines. Their key activities are summarized in Table 1.

■ The advent of sophisticated molecular technology has allowed the generation of highly specific molecular antagonists to cytokines. These "biological therapies" may be (i) monoclonal antibodies (e.g. infliximab, adalimumab); (ii) native cytokine receptors coupled to the Fc component of human

Table 1 Major biological effects of the pro-inflammatory cytokines TNFα and IL-1β

Cell	Effect	Clinical consequence
Macrophage	Cytokine production	Perpetuation of inflammation
Lymphocyte	T-cell activation	Perpetuation of inflammation
Endothelial cell	Activation, adhesion molecule expression	Recruitment of leucocytes to joints
Fibroblast	Enzyme release (e.g. MMP, prostaglandin synthesis)	Tissue degradation
Chondrocyte	Matrix breakdown	Tissue degradation
Osteoclast	Maturation/activation	Bone erosion

immunoglobulin (e.g. etanercept); or (iii) natural antagonists that closely resemble the cytokine structure, but deliver no signal when bound by receptor (e.g. anakinra).

This chapter addresses the clinical utility of agents that specifically block TNFα and IL-1 activities in inflammatory arthritis.

■ ETANERCEPT

KEY INDICATIONS

- Rheumatoid arthritis
- Psoriatic arthritis (US licence only)
- Juvenile inflammatory arthritis

Evidence for benefit

Four randomized, controlled double-blind trials provide the core evidence for benefit in rheumatoid arthritis (RA). These are summarized in Table 2. Monotherapy promotes benefit at the ACR 20 level in around 60–70% of recipients within 8–12 weeks with progressively smaller numbers achieving significant improvement at ACR 50 and ACR 70 levels, respectively. Benefit has been shown in reduced clinical inflammation, improved functional and quality of life indices and in reduced radiographic progression. In general withdrawal rates from studies favour etanercept over placebo.

The pivotal phase III study compared methotrexate with etanercept monotherapy in RA patients with less than three years' disease duration (Bathon 2000). Both therapeutic arms improved significantly by clinical response criteria and by reduced radiographic progression. Etanercept recipients exhibited marginal but nevertheless significantly greater improvement after one year than methotrexate recipients judged by ACR responses and Sharp erosion scores. Symptomatic control was evident at an earlier stage. In a further study, clinical benefit has also been shown when etanercept was used in combination with methotrexate following addition to partial or nonresponders to methotrexate (Weinblatt et al. 1999a).

Fewer studies have supported its use in other inflammatory diseases states. One randomized controlled study has reported benefit in psoriatic arthritis (see Table 3). Similarly, one controlled study reports benefit in ankylosing spondylitis. In all clinical indications, the longevity of clinical response and dropout rates in clinical practice are unclear.

Evidence for harm

Adverse events in randomized controlled trials were in general of a similar nature and frequency in etanercept compared with placebo recipients. In the pivotal phase III study 93% of etanercept recipients completed to one year; 5% discontinued because of an adverse event. Injection site reactions are associated

Table 2 Major randomized controlled trials for etanercept in rheumatoid arthritis

References	n	Comparator drugs	Study design	Study duration	Outcome efficacy	Outcome toxicity	Comment
Moreland et al. 1997	180	Etanercept (0.25, 2 and 16 mg/m²) vs placebo	RCT, DB SC injection	3 months	Etanercept (16 mg/m²) ACR 20—75% ACR 50—57% Significantly greater response than placebo	Similar to placebo	Early demonstration of efficacy
Weinblatt et al. 1999a	89	MTX + placebo vs MTX + etanercept 25 mg, twice weekly	RCT, DB SC injection	6 months	ACR 20—71 ACR 50—39 ACR 70—15 Significantly greater response than placebo	Injection site reactions greater in etanercept group. Other AE similar	Effective in partial MTX responders in combination with MTX
Moreland et al. 1999	234	Placebo vs etanercept 10 mg/twice weekly vs etanercept 25 mg/twice weekly	RCT, DB SC injection	6 months	ACR 20—59 ACR 50—40 ACR 70—15 Significantly greater response than placebo	Similar to placebo	Effective monotherapy
Bathon et al. 2000 (ERA)	632	MTX vs etanercept 10 mg/twice weekly v etanercept 25 mg/twice weekly	RCT, DB SC injection	12 months	ACRn greater in etanercept than MTX group. ACR 20, 50 70 at 12 months similar in etanercept vs MTX groups. Etanercept associated with superior erosion. Retardation at 12 months	Similar to MTX in general. Trend to reduced infection rate compared with MTX group	Demonstrates marginal but significant superiority to MTX as monotherapy in early (<3 years) RA

Table 3 Clinical studies supporting use of TNF-targeting agents in seronegative arthropathies

Drug	Reference/disease	n	Comparator drugs	Study design	Study duration	Outcome efficacy	Outcome, toxicity	Comment
Etanercept	Mease et al. 2000 Psoriatic arthritis	60	Etanercept 25 mg SC twice weekly vs placebo	RCT, DB SC injection	12 weeks	87% etanercept met PsARC response vs 23% placebo recipients. PASI improved in some patients	Similar to placebo	Suggests etanercept has efficacy in psoriatic arthritis. Beneficial effect in skin component also but limited sample population
Etanercept	Gorman et al. 2002 Ankylosing spondylitis (AS)	40	Etanercept 25 mg SC twice weekly vs placebo	RCT, DB SC injection	4 months	80% achieved treatment response vs 30% in placebo recipients (Assessments in AS Working Group)	Similar to placebo	Effective in AS. Possible effects in spinal disease of interest
Infliximab	Braun et al. 2002 Ankylosing spondylitis	70	Infliximab IV 5 mg/kg vs placebo	RCT, DB, multi-centre	12 weeks	53% infliximab recipients achieved 50% improvement in BASDAI vs 9% given placebo	Infliximab recipients: episode of TB, allergic granulomatosis and transient leucopenia	Efficacy demonstrated—caution expressed regarding potential immunosuppression

PsARC, psoriatic arthritis response criteria; PASI, psoriasis area and severity index; BASDAI, Bath ankylosing spondylitis disease activity index.

with etanercept use (37% in trials), but rarely caused drug cessation. They usually occur in the first month and reduce thereafter. Only preliminary post-marketing surveillance data are as yet available and frequency estimates of toxic events are unknown. Allergic reactions to etanercept are rare (<0.5%). Minor (~20%) and major infections (~1%) are similar to rates in placebo recipients in controlled trials. Rates of malignancies in treated patients are similar to those expected as predicted by national epidemiology database. Post-marketing reports have highlighted risks of reactivation of tuberculosis, demyelination and blood dyscrasias. Patients with demyelinating disease should not receive etanercept.

Prescribing etanercept

Practical guidelines for prescribing are shown in Table 4. BSR guidelines on eligibility for etanercept therapy are shown at www.rheumatology.org.uk (guidelines). *Efficacy should be monitored* three-monthly according to the BSR guidelines using the disease activity score (DAS). Therapy should be withdrawn after three months if there is a lack of response. Response is defined as DAS28 improvement by >1.2, or achievement of DAS28 <3.2.

Drug interactions

None have been reported.

■ INFLIXIMAB

KEY INDICATIONS

■ Rheumatoid arthritis (combination with methotrexate)

Evidence for benefit

Two randomized, controlled double-blind trials provide the core evidence for benefit of infliximab in RA. These are summarized in Table 5. Monotherapy with infliximab in early studies indicated propensity to antichimeric antibody formation, which may enhance clearance and thereby interfere with function. Clinical use is indicated, therefore, in combination with methotrexate (MTX). Infliximab and low-dose MTX promote benefit at the ACR 20 level in around 60% of recipients within 8–12 weeks with progressively smaller numbers achieving significant improvement at ACR 50 and ACR 70 levels, respectively. Benefit has been shown in reduced clinical inflammation, improved functional and quality of life indices and in reduced radiographic progression.

The pivotal phase III study compared MTX/placebo with MTX/infliximab (four dose regimens) in combination in RA patients with mean disease duration of 9–12 years and in whom an inadequate response to MTX therapy had been obtained. MTX/infliximab recipients exhibited significantly greater improvement

Table 4 Prescribing guidelines for etanercept

Pharmacology	TNF receptor (p75) dimer, Fc fusion protein Half-life 115 hours	No data on overdosage
Dose	25 mg twice weekly, 1 ml SC self injection	Rotate injection site ISR commonest in first month—usually self resolving
Contraindications	Pregnancy, breast feeding, ongoing active infection, chronic leg ulcers, previous TB without appropriate treatment, septic arthritis (<12 months), septic prosthesis (as long as it remains *in situ*), recurrent chest infection, indwelling urinary catheter, multiple sclerosis, malignancy or premalignant states (excluding basal cell carcinoma, malignancies diagnosed and treated >10 years ago)	Limited clinical experience with this drug class
Cautions	ANA positivity	May be used in combination with MTX, glucocorticoids, NSAIDs, simple analgesics (e.g. paracetamol). Not to be combined with anakinra. Risk in ANA-positive RA patients of CT overlap appears low but caution advised
Monitoring		Recommend FBC monthly for three months then two monthly
Vaccination	Live vaccines should **not** be administered	No information on effect of etanercept on killed vaccine efficacy
Screening	CXR, FBC, biochemistry profile, ANA	TB screening—CXR, skin testing according to local guidelines
Eligibility	Active RA—DAS.5.1 on two occasions one month apart	BSR guidelines define criteria
Alcohol	National guidelines apply	
Pregnancy	Avoid	Insufficient data available in human subjects. No evidence of harm in rodents
Breast feeding	Avoid	Insufficient data available

Table 5 Major randomized controlled trials for infliximab in rheumatoid arthritis

References	n	Comparator drugs	Study design	Study duration	Outcome efficacy	Outcome, toxicity	Comment
Maini et al. (1998)	101	Infliximab/MTX vs Infliximab/placebo vs MTX/placebo	RCT, DB IV infusion	26 weeks	60% infliximab/MTX recipients achieved 20% Paulus response	Well tolerated. Similar to placebo	Early demonstration of efficacy
Maini et al. (1999) (ATTRACT)	428	MTX/placebo vs MTX plus one of: Infliximab 3 mg/kg—8 weeks Infliximab 3 mg/kg—4 weeks Infliximab 10 mg/kg—8 weeks Infliximab 10 mg/kg—4 weeks	RCT, DB IV infusion	30 weeks	Infliximab 3 mg/kg/MTX ACR 20—50 ACR 50—27 ACR 70—8 Significantly greater response than placebo/MTX	Similar to placebo. ANA positive greater in infliximab-treated groups	Effective in partial MTX responders in combination with MTX
Lipsky et al. (2000) (ATTRACT)	428	MTX/placebo vs MTX plus one of: Infliximab 3 mg/kg—8 weeks Infliximab 3 mg/kg—4 weeks Infliximab 10 mg/kg—8 weeks Infliximab 10 mg/kg—4 weeks	RCT, DB IV infusion	54 weeks	Infliximab 3 mg/kg/MTX ACR 20—42 ACR 50—21 ACR 70—10 Significantly greater response than placebo/MTX. Significant retardation of radiographic progression	Similar to placebo	Effective therapy in combination with MTX

after one year than MTX/placebo recipients judged by higher ACR 20, ACR 50 and ACR 70 response rates and reduced progression of Sharp score. No progression in radiographic joint destruction was observed even in "clinical nonresponders" in MTX/infliximab recipients groups.

Fewer studies support its use in other inflammatory diseases states. Two controlled studies have reported benefit in ankylosing spondylitis. These are summarized in Table 3. No controlled studies are yet reported in psoriatic arthritis, although controlled data indicate efficacy in psoriasis. Open-label evidence supports efficacy in only psoriatic arthritis thus far. In all clinical indications, the longevity of the clinical response and dropout rates in practice are unclear.

Evidence for harm

Adverse events in randomized controlled trials were in general of a similar nature and frequency in infliximab/MTX compared with placebo/MTX recipients. In the pivotal phase III study 73% of infliximab (3 mg/kg)/MTX recipients completed to one year; 6% discontinued because of an adverse event. Only preliminary post-marketing surveillance data are as yet available, and therefore frequency estimates of toxic events are unknown. Allergic reactions to infliximab are rare (<0.1%). Urticaria, dyspnoea and hypotension associated with infusion have been reported (appropriate resuscitation drugs and facilities should be available). Minor (up to 34%) and major infections (~2–8%) are statistically similar to rates in placebo recipients in controlled trials. However, trends to increased frequency of urinary tract infections, pharyngitis and sinusitis have been observed in infliximab recipients. Rates of malignancies in treated patients are similar to those expected as predicted by the NEER database. Post-marketing reports have highlighted the risk of reactivation of tuberculosis (usually within three months of commencing therapy; they may be extrapulmonary), demyelination and blood dyscrasias. Patients with demyelinating disease should not receive infliximab. A recent study in patients with congestive cardiac failure indicated cardiac function deterioration in infliximab recipients. Infliximab should not be given to patients with NYHA class III/IV cardiac failure.

Prescribing infliximab

Practical guidelines for prescribing are shown in Table 6. BSR guidelines on eligibility for infliximab therapy are shown at www.rheumatology.org.uk (guidelines). Efficacy should be monitored three-monthly as per BSR guidelines using the DAS. Therapy should be withdrawn after three months if there is a lack of response. Response is defined as DAS28 improvement by >1.2, or achievement of DAS28 <3.2.

Drug interactions

None have been reported. There is possible cross-reactivity with other chimaeric monoclonal antibodies (e.g. anti-CD4 monoclonal antibodies).

Table 6   Prescribing guidelines for infliximab

Pharmacology	Chimeric murine/human monoclonal anti-TNFα antibody	No data on overdosage
Dose	Flush line with 50 ml 0.9% saline, then 3 mg/kg given IV over at least 2 hours (2ml/min max). Dose administered week 0, week 2, week 6 and 8 weekly thereafter. MTX to continue as previously prescribed. Folic acid 5 mg/week to continue as previously prescribed	Monitor vital signs every 30 minutes. Open studies suggest some patients require increased dose (to 5mg/kg) or reduced frequency of administration (to six weekly) to maintain response
Contraindications	Pregnancy, breast feeding, ongoing active infection, chronic leg ulcers, previous TB without appropriate treatment, septic arthritis (<12 months), septic prosthesis (as long as remains *in situ*), recurrent chest infection, indwelling urinary catheter, multiple sclerosis, malignancy or pre-malignant states (excluding basal cell carcinoma, malignancies diagnosed and treated >10 years ago), cardiac failure (NYHA class III/IV)	Limited clinical experience with this drug class
Cautions	ANA positivity	Must be used in combination with MTX. May be used together with glucocorticoids, NSAIDs, simple analgesics (e.g. paracetamol). Not to be combined with anakinra. Risk in ANA-positive RA patients of CT overlap appears low, but caution advised
Monitoring	As per MTX monitoring recommendations (page 63)	
Vaccination	Live vaccines should **not** be administered	No information on effect of infliximab on killed vaccine efficacy
Screening	CXR, FBC, biochemistry profile, ANA	TB screening—CXR, skin testing according to local guidelines
Eligibility	Active RA—DAS.5.1 on two occasions one month apart	BSR guidelines define criteria
Alcohol	Guidelines apply with respect to concomitant MTX	
Pregnancy	Avoid	Insufficient data available in human subjects. No evidence of harm in rodents
Breast feeding	Avoid	Insufficient data available

■ ADALIMUMAB (D2E7)

KEY INDICATIONS
- Rheumatoid arthritis

Evidence for benefit
Several randomised, controlled double blind trials provide the core evidence for benefit in rheumatoid arthritis (RA), either as monotherapy or in combination with methotrexate (see Table 7). Most data are available at the time of publication only in abstract form – one phase II study has been published (ARMADA; Weinblatt 2003). This pivotal, 24 week phase II study compared placebo / MTX with adalimumab (20 mg, 40 mg or 80 mg every other week s.c.) / MTX in combination in RA patients (n = 271) with range of mean disease duration 11–13 years and in whom an inadequate response to MTX therapy had been obtained. Adalimumab/MTX recipients exhibited significantly greater improvement after 24 weeks than placebo/MTX recipients judged by higher ACR20 (67% vs 15%), ACR50 (55% vs 8%) and ACR70 (27% vs 5%) response rates (response rates shown for 40 mg e.o.w./MTX vs placebo/MTX). Suppression of serum proMMP1 and proMMP3 (possible surrogates for radiographic progression) was observed. Abstract presentations (ACR Scientific Meeting 2002) report suppression of progression in radiographic joint destruction in adalimumab recipients compared with controls. Reported data also demonstrate improvements in quality of life/physical function and fatigue scores with adalimumab.

Evidence for harm
Adverse events in randomised controlled trials were in general of similar nature and frequency in adalimumab compared with placebo recipients. Only preliminary surveillance data are as yet available and as such frequency estimates of toxic events are unknown. Injection site reactions are reported in approximately 20% of recipients in trials vs 14% placebo. However, trends to increased frequency of URTI, pharyngitis and sinusitis have been observed in other TNF-blocked recipients and there is no reason as yet to differentiate adalimumab from other products. Similarly, concerns about tuberculosis infection remain across this class of agents and adequate screening is necessary as required by local guidelines. No alteration in cancer rates was evident compared with those expected in the population. Antibodies against adalimumab have been detected in 5.5% of patients and have not as yet been associated with harm or effect on efficacy.

Prescribing adalimumab
Adalimumab has not yet been licensed at the time of publication. (US FDA approval was granted 31 December 2002.) As such a table of prescribing guidelines is not yet possible. The reader is referred to the appropriate prescribers' informa-

Table 7 Major randomised controlled trials for adalimumab in rheumatoid arthritis

References	n	Comparator drugs	Study design	Study duration	Outcome efficacy	Outcome toxicity	Comment
Weinblatt et al. 2003	271	MTX/Adalinumab (20 mg eow, 40 mg eow, 80 mg eow) vs MTX/placebo	RCT, DB, SC injection	24 weeks	Adalimumab 40 mg eow ACR20 – 67.2% ACR50 – 55.2% ACR70 – 26.9% Significantly greater response than placebo	Injection site reaction greater in adalimumab group, 0.28 per patient-year vs 0.09	Suggests adalimumab 40 mg eow as appropriate dose, with sustained results and rapid onset of action
Keystone et al. ACR 2002 (abstract 468)	619	MTX/Adalimumab (20 mg weekly, 40 mg eow) vs MTX/placebo	RCT, DB, SC injection	52 weeks	Adalimumab 40 mg eow ACR20 – 58.9% ACR50 – 41.5% ACR70 – 23.2% Adalimumab/MTX was significantly better than placebo/MTX at inhibiting erosions and joint space narrowing. Patients with no new erosions at 52 weeks adalimumab/MTX, 61.8% vs 46% Significantly greater response than placebo	Overall incidence of adverse events was consistent with the general RA population	Effective in treating signs and symptoms of RA and inhibiting radiographic disease progression.
van de Putte et al. ACR 2002 (abstract 467)	544	Adalimumab 20 mg weekly, 20 mg eow, 40 mg weekly, 40 mg eow) vs placebo	RCT, DB, SC injection	26 week	Adalimumab 40 mg eow ACR20 – 46% ACR50 – 22.1% ACR70 – 12.4% Adalimumab 40 mg weekly ACR20 – 53.4% ACR50 – 35% ACR70 – 18.4% Significantly greater response than placebo	Adalimumab was generally well tolerated compared to placebo. Most common adverse events possibly related to the study drug were injection-site reactions (9.7%), rash (9.4%), and headache (9.4%).	Adalimumab monotherapy demonstrated rapid and consistent efficacy in treating the signs and symptoms of RA. Some patients may benefit from an increase in dose to 40 mg adalimumab weekly
Furst et al. ACR 2002 (abstract 1537)	636	Adalimumab 40 mg eow/SOC vs placebo/SOC Patients were randomised to receive adalimumab or placebo in combination with SOC (standard of care; other DMARDs, steroids, NSAIDs). Other DMARDs used: methotrexate (59.3%), antimalarials (24.7%), leflunomide (13.4%), sulfasalazine (9.7%), parenteral gold (5.8%)	RCT, DB, SC injection	24 weeks	Adalimumab 40 mg eow ACR20 – 51.9% ACR50 – 28.9% ACR70 – 14.8% Significantly greater response than placebo	Similar to placebo in terms of any AE, SAE, infections, serious infections	Adalimumab is well tolerated and efficacious when given in RA in addition to multiple other antirheumatic therapies

tion. Adalimumab is anticipated to be administered at 40 mg e.o.w. by s.c. injection either as monotherapy or in combination with MTX. In monotherapy, some patients may benefit from an increase in dose to 40 mg adalimumab weekly. Eligibility for adalimumab is anticipated to be the same as for other TNF blockers and relevant BSR guidelines are shown at www.rheumatology.org.uk (guidelines). *Efficacy should be monitored* 3-monthly as per BSR guidelines using the DAS. Therapy should be withdrawn after 3 months if there is lack of response. Response is defined as DAS28 improvement by >1.2, or achievement of DAS28 <3.2.

Drug interactions
None reported.

■ ANAKINRA (IL-1Ra)

KEY INDICATIONS
■ Rheumatoid arthritis

Evidence for benefit
Two published, peer reviewed, randomized, controlled double-blind trials provide the core evidence for benefit in RA. These are summarized in Table 8. Monotherapy promotes benefit at the ACR 20 level in around 40% of recipients within 8–12 weeks with significantly fewer achieving significant improvement at ACR 50 and ACR 70 levels. Combination of anakinra with MTX also offers benefit in comparison with MTX/placebo, suggesting that anakinra may also offer benefit in DMARD partial or nonresponders. Benefit has been shown in reduced clinical inflammation, in improved functional and quality of life indices and in reduced radiographic progression.

The pivotal phase III study compared methotrexate/placebo with MTX/anakinra in RA patients with median 6.5–8.8 years' disease duration in whom a partial response or no response to MTX was achieved. Addition of anakinra (1 mg/kg) brought about significant improvement compared with addition of placebo as measured by clinical response criteria (42% ACR 20 response compared with 23% in placebo recipients).

No studies as yet support its use in other inflammatory diseases states. In all clinical indications, the longevity of the clinical response and dropout rates in clinical practice are unclear. Long-term safety studies evaluating anakinra are underway.

Evidence for harm
Adverse events in randomized controlled trials were in general of a similar nature and frequency in anakinra compared with placebo recipients. In the pivotal phase III study 78% of anakinra recipients completed to six months;

Table 8 Major randomized controlled trials for anakinra (Kineret) in rheumatoid arthritis

References	n	Comparator drugs	Study design	Study duration	Outcome efficacy	Outcome, toxicity	Comment
Bresnihan et al. (1998)	472	Placebo vs Anakinra 30 mg/day vs Anakinra 75 mg/day vs Anakinra 150 mg/day	RCT, DB SC injection	24 weeks	Anakinra 150 mg/day ACR 20—43% ACR 50—19% ACR 70—1% Radiographic progression reduced by anakinra (Larsen, and erosion count)	ISR common in anakinra groups. Other AE reported similar to placebo	Early indication of potential efficacy, particularly in radiographic progression
Cohen et al. (2002)	419	MTX/placebo vs MTX plus one of: Anakinra 0.04 mg/kg Anakinra 0.1 mg/kg Anakinra 0.4 mg/kg Anakinra 1.0 mg/kg Anakinra 2.0 mg/kg	RCT, DB SC injection	24 weeks	Anakinra 1 mg/kg ACR 20—42% ACR 50—24% ACR 70—10% Significantly greater response than placebo/MTX	Similar to placebo. Increase ISR	Effective in partial MTX responders in combination with MTX
Jiang et al. (2000)	472	Placebo vs Anakinra 30 mg/day vs Anakinra 75 mg/day vs Anakinra 150 mg/day	RCT, DB SC injection	48 weeks	Anakinra reduced radiographic progression—Larsen or Genant methods	N/A	Confirms capacity to modify radiographic progression
Amgen study 1 access via Amgen website	501	Placebo/MTX vs Anakinra 100mg/day/ MTX	RCT, DB SC injection	24 weeks	Anakinra 100 mg/day ACR 20—38% ACR 50—17% ACR 70—6% Significantly greater response than placebo/MTX	Not shown	

13.6% discontinued because of an adverse event. Injection site reactions have been associated with anakinra use (>60% in trials), and although these were mostly of mild to moderate severity, they did cause withdrawal in 7% of recipients. The severity of injection site reactions was reduced with treatment cycle. Only preliminary post-marketing surveillance data are as yet available, and therefore frequency estimates of toxic events are unknown. Allergic reactions to anakinra are rare (<0.5%). Minor (~30%, especially upper respiratory) and major infections (~2%) are slightly more common than in placebo recipients in controlled trials. A recent open study has suggested increased risk of serious infection when anakinra and TNF blocking agents were used in combination. There may be greater risk in asthmatic patients. Rates of malignancy in treated patients are similar to those expected as predicted by the NEER database. Neutropenia has been occasionally observed.

Prescribing anakinra

Practical guidelines for prescribing are shown in Table 9. BSR guidelines on eligibility for anakinra therapy are available at www.rheumatology.org.uk (guidelines). *Efficacy should be monitored* three-monthly as per BSR guidelines for TNF blockers using the DAS. Therapy should be withdrawn after three months if there is a lack of response. Response is defined as DAS28 improvement by >1.2, or achievement of DAS28 <3.2.

Drug interactions

None has been reported. Note the predominant renal clearance.

■ COMMON ISSUES FOR BIOLOGICAL THERAPIES

Registry issues

Subsequent to obtaining informed consent from patients, all recipients of cytokine-inhibitory agents should be submitted to the BSR registry, together with clinical information entered by proforma. Information can be obtained from the BSR website at www.rheumatology.org.uk. Control patients are also being entered from selected clinical centres. This will ensure long-term identification of efficacy and safety as clinical experience is acquired.

Table 9 Prescribing guidelines for anakinra

Pharmacology	Recombinant IL-1Ra Half-life 4-6 hours	No data on overdosage
Dose	100 mg/day—self administered SC injection of 1ml clear solution	ISR common. Plasma clearance reduced by 75% if creatinine clearance <30 ml/min. Do not use if particulate material in vial. Store at 4°C
Contraindications	Known hypersensitivity to E. coli-derived products, pregnancy, breast feeding, ongoing active infection, chronic leg ulcers, previous TB without appropriate treatment, septic arthritis (<12 months), septic prosthesis (as long as it remains in situ), recurrent chest infection, malignancy or premalignant states (excluding basal cell carcinoma, malignancies diagnosed and treated >10 years ago), persistent neutropenia	Limited clinical experience with this drug class
Cautions		May be used together with MTX, glucocorticoids, NSAIDs, simple analgesics (e.g. paracetamol). **Not** to be used with TNF blocking agents
Monitoring	FBC monthly for three months then quarterly thereafter	As per MTX monitoring recommendations (page 63) if on combination
Vaccination	Live vaccines should **not** be administered	No information on effect of anakinra on killed vaccine efficacy
Screening	CXR, FBC, biochemistry profile, ANA	TB screening—CXR, skin testing according to local guidelines
Eligibility	Active RA—DAS.5.1 on two occasions one month apart	
Alcohol	National guidelines apply	
Pregnancy	Avoid	Insufficient data available in human subjects. No. evidence of harm in rodents
Breast feeding	Avoid	Insufficient data available

NICE recommendations

The National Institute for Clinical Excellence (NICE) offered detailed recommendations for the use of TNF blocking agents in March 2002. The Health Technology Board in Scotland ratified these recommendations in May 2002. Key guidance for use of TNF blocking agents as follows:

1. Recommended for active RA and having failed at least two previous DMARDs (to include MTX unless contraindicated).
2. Should follow BSR guidelines, April 2001.
3. Should be prescribed by a consultant rheumatologist specializing in their use. Choice of agent by specific discussion between physician and patient.
4. Maintenance therapy at lowest licensed effective dose.
5. With patients' consent, all recipients to be include in BSR registry.
6. No evidence to support treatment beyond four years at this time.
7. No evidence for consecutive use of TNF blocking agents, and this is not recommended.

Anakinra (IL-1Ra) has not yet been reviewed by NICE. Details available at www.nice.org.uk or telephone 0870 1555 455.

KEY REFERENCES

■ Updated Consensus Statement 2001

■ Bathon *et al.* 2000

■ Lipsky *et al.* 2000

■ Weinblatt *et al.* 2003

■ Cohen *et al.* 2002

■ USEFUL SOURCES OF INFORMATION

■ National Institute for Clinical Excellence, NICE – www.nice.org.uk
■ Federal Drug Administration – www.fda.gov
■ British Society for Rheumatology – www.rheumatology.org.uk

■ Combination therapy: conventional DMARDs

Single, sequential DMARDs seldom induce remission. As patient and physician expectation of desired response in rheumatoid arthritis (RA) has increased, so combinations have been used more widely. The evidence base for the majority of regimens is minimal.

■ Combination options
Step-up regimens may appear the most logical, since some patients will do well on a single agent. Nevertheless, step-down and parallel strategies have also been employed in a number of studies (see Table 1).

■ Toxicity issues
An unresolved practical issue is how to decide which therapy to stop when a patient on combination therapy develops an adverse event which might occur with either (e.g. leucopenia or abnormal liver function tests). The pragmatic approach is to stop both drugs, then re-introduce the one first used, or the one best tolerated from other points of view in that patient.

■ Evidence base
A summary of major combination studies of conventional DMARDs is shown in Table 1. The meta-analysis (Felson 1994) concluded that combination therapy did not offer substantial benefit in terms of efficacy, and toxicity was increased.

Since that meta-analysis there have been six parallel (five blind, one open) one step-up and two step-down studies using conventional DMARDs. Apart from the studies of Tugwell and the two studies from O'Dell utilizing triple therapy with hydroxychloroquine, methotrexate and sulphasalazine, the results have been disappointing. A number of other studies are currently being conducted and results are awaited.

A study of the bioavailability of methotrexate in the presence of HCQ showed that the AUC for MTX was increased and maximum MTX concentrations decreased when MTX was co-administered with HCQ (Carmichael 2002). The results may explain the potency of MTX-HCQ combinations. Authors suggest extra vigilance for MTX adverse effects during MTX-HCQ combination, especially if renal function is impaired.

Table 1 Selected combination studies of conventional DMARDs

Author	Year	Intervention	n	Strategy	Outcome	Comment
Porter	1993	IM gold 6/12 suboptimal response →HCQ/placebo	440	Step up double-blind RCT	Efficacy: no Toxicity: no increase	No justification for combination gold + HCQ in patients with partial response to gold
Tugwell	1995	Cyclosporin + MTX vs placebo + MTX over 6/12	148	Step up double-blind RCT	Efficacy: increased with combination Side-effects 'not substantially increased'	Patients on combination improved Long-term follow-up needed
O'Dell	1996	MTX SASP + HCQ MTX + SASP + HCQ over 2 years	102	Parallel double-blind RCT	Efficacy: triple better than dual or mono Toxicity: no increase	77% of triple group achieved 50% improvement at 9/12 and maintained to 2 years
Boers	1997	SASP vs SASP + MTX + prednisolone 60mg (tapered)	155	Step down double-blind RCT	Efficacy: combination therapy better than mono Toxicity: fewer withdrawals in combined group	Confirmatory studies and long-term follow-up needed
Haagsma	1997	SASP vs MTX vs SASP + MTX combination over 1 year	105	Parallel double-blind RCT	Efficacy: no differences between 3 treatment arms Toxicity: nausea more often in combination. Withdrawals = 3 groups	Results of MTX, SASP and combination very comparable
Dougados	1997	SASP vs MTX vs combination over 1 year	209	Parallel RCT	Efficacy: clinical and radiological benefit similar in all 3 groups Toxicity: nausea more common with combination	No clinically relevant benefit of combination
Möttönen	1999	Single drug vs SASP MTX HCQ and prednisolone over 2 years	199	Step down RCT	Efficacy: ACR 50 in 58% single drug and 71% in combination p=0.058 Toxicity: similar	Combination not more hazardous ?Better in a proportion of patients
Proudman	2000	SASP vs MTX, cyclosporin and intra-articular steroids 48 weeks	82	Parallel RCT	Efficacy: similar clinical and radiological Toxicity: hypertension and renal in combination group	More rapid improvement in combination but ACR and remission rates not better Suggest step up approach may be better
O'Dell	2002	MTX + HCQ MTX + SASP MTX + HCQ + SASP over 2 years	171	Parallel double-blind RCT	Efficacy: ACR 20 improvement greatest with triple therapy 78% Toxicity: all combination well tolerated	Efficacy of triple therapy is superior to double combination used in this trial
Gerards	2003	CsA + MTX vs CsA + placebo over 48 weeks	120	Parallel double-blind RCT	Efficacy: combination probably better than CsA alone Toxicity: tendency to greater toxicity in combination groups	Neither therapy effective in inducing remission. Combination better in slowing radiological progression. Cyclosporin monotherapy should be compared with methotrexate monotherapy

4 CORTICOSTEROIDS

Since the inception of their use in rheumatoid arthritis (RA) (Hench *et al.* 1949), corticosteroids have remained one of the most powerful therapeutic options available. They are widely used in routine clinical practice but their place in the management of RA remains the subject of debate (Dennison and Cooper 1998; Laan *et al.* 1999; Boers 1999) and controversy (Morrison and Capell 1999; Conn 2002; Saag 2001; Edwards *et al.* 2002) as clinicians and patients alike remain concerned about both short- and long-term adverse effects.

Corticosteroids can be delivered:

- Locally, as intra-articular (IA) injections
- Systemically by the oral, intramuscular (IM) or intravenous (IV) routes

Corticosteroids administered locally and systemically are often used in combination with conventional disease-modifying antirheumatic drugs (DMARDs) at a time of marked disease activity or perhaps to bridge the lag interval between the introduction of a DMARD and the onset of clinical improvement. Guidelines for their use in the treatment of extra-articular manifestations of RA (e.g. vasculitis, interstitial lung disease) or in the treatment of DMARD adverse effects (e.g. aurothiomalate-induced thrombocytopenia) are not included. The aim of this chapter is to provide a practical guide to the use of corticosteroids in the management of the articular manifestations of RA in routine clinical practice.

■ LOCAL (IA) CORTICOSTEROID

IA injections of corticosteroid are widely used to give rapid symptomatic relief to actively synovitic joints. Clinical trials with regard to long-term effects on radiographic progression and disability are not practical within current strategies advocated for the treatment of RA. IA injections have traditionally been undertaken by doctors but are increasingly being performed by other members of the multidisciplinary team, including nurses and physiotherapists.

KEY INDICATIONS FOR INTRA-ARTICULAR STEROIDS

- Pain relief, especially when only one or a few joints are inflamed
- Local treatment of synovitic joints whilst minimizing adverse systemic effects
- Rapid symptom control pending the onset of DMARD effect
- Problem joints treated when overall disease control is good

---

Injection technique

General principles only are considered here, as detailed accounts of techniques for the injection of specific joints are well covered elsewhere (Doherty *et al.* 1992; Seror *et al.* 1999).

- *Aseptic precautions.* IA joint injection is carried out using careful aseptic precautions or a no-touch technique in order to minimize the risk of introducing infection. If these techniques are observed, the risk of infection is small (Jones *et al.* 1993).
- *Use of ultrasound.* Most rheumatologists carry out IA injection after clinical examination and identification of bony landmarks. However, this can be inaccurate, reducing the beneficial response achieved (Grassi *et al.* 1999). Therefore, there has been growing interest in the use of ultrasound-guided IA joint injection to improve accuracy, especially for small joint injection (Balint *et al.* 2002; Weitoft and Uddenfeldt 2002).
- *Synovial fluid aspirate.* Synovial fluid aspiration prior to injection of steroid is thought to lower the risk of relapse in that joint and is recommended (Fitzgerald *et al.* 1985). Whether joint washout with saline confers additional benefit is less clear (Srinivasan *et al.* 1995; Chakravarty *et al.* 1994) and it is not part of our routine practice. If there is any clinical suspicion that a joint is infected or the synovial fluid appears turbid, Gram stain and culture are essential and injection with corticosteroid should not be undertaken. If the clinical suspicion is high, treatment with antibiotics should be started immediately.
- *Post-injection rest.* Post-injection rest for 24 hours has been shown to be beneficial in terms of the duration of the clinical response (BNF 2002). However, as the majority of IA injections are carried out in the out-patient department, this may not be practical. A reasonable compromise is to advise the patient to rest the joint as much as possible at home in the 24 hours after injection.

Choice of corticosteroid preparation

Corticosteroids with a long-acting depot effect are preferred for IA joint injection (e.g. triamcinolone acetonide) (Empire Rheumatism Council 1957), but there are few studies of the various preparations available (Blyth *et al.* 1994). Frequent requirement for joint injection should prompt a review of the patient's DMARD therapy.

Complications of IA corticosteroid injection

Complications associated with this procedure are shown in Table 1. Clinically significant adverse events are rare.

Cautions
- Diabetic patients—diabetic control may be affected temporarily.
- Anticoagulated patients—extra care is needed when injecting large joints, small joint injection not recommended. Worth checking INR beforehand.

Table 1	Complications of IA corticosteroid injection

1. Short-term facial flushing
2. Increased pain in the joint for 24 hours after injection. (Microcyrstaline suspension of steroid may give rise to a crystal synovitis)
3. Septic arthritis
4. Skin/muscle atrophy at the injection site

Contraindications
■ Infection in the joint, skin or systemically.

Post-injection advice to patient
■ Short-lasting facial flushing may occur
■ Joint may be painful up to 24 hours after the injection
■ Joint should be rested as much as possible for 24 hours
■ May take several days for benefit to occur
■ Contact number of specialist unit given, should problems arise

---

Summary
■ IA delivery of corticosteroid is a safe and effective way to provide rapid symptom relief when one or a few joints only are affected.
■ Local treatment also minimizes adverse systemic effects.

■ SYSTEMIC CORTICOSTEROIDS IN THE TREATMENT OF RA

■ Oral
■ Intramuscular (IM) and intravenous (IV)

Oral corticosteroids
The optimal use of oral corticosteroids in the treatment of RA is still the subject of much debate. The development of clear guidelines is hampered by the lack of large randomized controlled trials. In this section their effect on disease activity and progression in RA will be reviewed.

Effect on disease activity
One of the first clinical trials was undertaken by the Empire Rheumatism Council (ERC) (1957) comparing the effects of cortisone and aspirin over three years. Patient well-being and function improved equally in both groups.

Erythrocyte sedimentation rate (ESR) decreased over the first two months in the cortisone group, but this effect had disappeared by six months. The group concluded that no definite additional benefit was obtained using corticosteroid.

Several recent meta-analyses have shown that low-dose corticosteroid administered for periods of approximately six months (and <1 year) improve disease activity indices and are effective in the short-term treatment of RA (Saff *et al.* 1996; Gotzsche and Myerson 1998; Criswell *et al.* 2002). Longer-term symptomatic benefit, however, is less certain. In a study of 128 patients with early RA randomized to either prednisolone 7.5 mg/day or placebo, in addition to NSAIDs and DMARDs over a two-year period, additional symptomatic benefit was shown in the prednisolone-treated patients, but this was not maintained beyond 6–9 months (Kirwan 1995).

In a study of oral corticosteroids as bridge therapy, 40 RA patients starting aurothioglucose were randomized to receive either prednisolone 10 mg/day or placebo for the first 12 weeks. During this period disease activity was significantly lower in the prednisolone group but a rebound deterioration occurred when the dose was tapered (van Gestel *et al.* 1995).

In a randomized comparison of combined prednisolone, methotrexate and sulphasalazine with sulphasalazine alone in 155 patients with early RA, clinical improvement was seen in both groups, but was significantly better in the combined group at 28 weeks. However, the clinical difference between the groups decreased and was no longer significant after prednisolone was stopped and there were no further changes when methotrexate was discontinued (Boers *et al.* 1997).

Therefore, whilst regular oral corticosteroid may confer short-term symptomatic relief and may be helpful as bridge therapy when starting a new DMARD, clinical benefit is not sustained in the longer term.

Effect on disease progression

The effect of corticosteroids on the progression of erosions in RA and thus the amount of joint destruction has been considered in a number of studies. Comparison between these is often problematic because of the variable disease duration in the patients included, differences in X-ray scoring systems, different trial durations and the small numbers of patients included in some studies.

In the ERC study of cortisone vs aspirin in the treatment of RA, both groups showed radiological deterioration. This was more marked in the aspirin group at two years, but the difference was not significant (Empire Rheumatism Council 1957). By contrast, the Medical Research Council (MRC) comparative study of high-dose prednisolone (initially 20 mg/day) and analgesics showed a reduction in the progression of erosions in the prednisolone group over two years (Joint Committee of the MRC 1960). In the third year of the trial, when the dose of prednisolone was lower (10 mg/day), radiological deterioration was roughly equal in both groups. The side-effect profile associated with the initial relatively high dose of prednisolone was considerable.

In a study of low-dose prednisolone treatment in early RA, Kirwan (1995) reported slowing both of radiological progression of disease and of the development of new erosions. The study was uncontrolled, however, for DMARD therapy; their contribution to the slowing of disease progression remains uncertain. In addition, in comparison with the treatment group at baseline, the placebo group contained a number of patients with more erosive disease. Whilst this progression did not reach significance, it would be important to know the X-ray progression of these particular patients. Subsequent follow-up one year after prednisolone withdrawal showed similar progression of erosive change in both groups (Hickling et al. 1998). Further follow-up of this cohort would be of interest, to assess whether early intervention with corticosteroids has an impact on disease outcome in the longer term.

In a recent study of step-down prednisolone (initially high dose and then reduced and stopped), methotrexate and sulphasalazine vs sulphasalazine alone in early RA, Boers et al. (1997) reported reduction in radiological progression in the combined group. However, the true effect of prednisolone here is difficult to extrapolate, owing to the combination of drugs. A methotrexate/sulphasalazine arm may have helped to answer this question.

Although interesting, these results need to be confirmed in further studies and their impact on longer-term disease outcome needs to be assessed, before the prescription of corticosteroids in early RA becomes routine.

■ IM AND IV CORTICOSTEROIDS IN THE TREATMENT OF RA

IM corticosteroids

Although often prescribed in RA to help settle a disease flare or as bridge therapy whilst awaiting the onset of action of conventional DMARDs, there are few studies assessing the effect of this therapy. In one study, 59 patients with RA commencing IM aurothiomalate were randomized to receive either three doses of IM depot methylprednisolone at 0, 4 and 8 weeks or matching placebo. The steroid-treated group showed more rapid improvement of symptoms at three months, but this additional benefit was not apparent at six months (Liebling et al. 1981). There are no data regarding effect on radiological progression.

IV corticosteroid

Several studies (Hansen et al. 1987, 1990; Ciconelli et al. 1996) have looked at the use of pulsed IV methylprednisolone (MP) in the treatment of RA. It is difficult, however, to draw any firm conclusions about the efficacy or toxicity of this form of therapy, as these studies involved small numbers of patients, were uncontrolled for DMARD therapy and used varying treatment regimens (e.g. IV MP daily for three days, IV MP monthly for six months) and MP dosage. Some studies have shown rapid symptom improvement in the MP-treated group (Hansen et al. 1987, 1990) whilst others have failed to demonstrate any difference (Ciconelli et al. 1996). No effect on radiological progression has been noted (Hansen *et al.* 1987, 1990; Ciconelli *et al.* 1996). There would therefore seem to be little indication for using this form of therapy.

■ ADVERSE EFFECTS OF SYSTEMIC CORTICOSTEROIDS

Since the earliest reports of steroid use in RA, clinicians and patients (Caldwell and Furst 1991; Leake 1995) alike have been concerned about their side-effect profile. The main adverse effects are shown in Table 2. Most organ systems can

Table 2	Adverse effects of systemic corticosteroids
System	*Adverse effect*
General	Weight gain Redistribution of body fat Infection Suppression of clinical signs of infection
Musculoskeletal	Osteoporosis/fracture Avascular necrosis Proximal myopathy Tendon rupture
Cutaneous	Acne Striae Hirsuitism Skin atrophy Bruising and purpura Impaired healing
Gastrointestinal	Dyspepsia Oesophageal ulceration and candidiasis Peptic ulceration (perforation) Acute pancreatitis
Cardiovascular	Fluid retention Hypertension Atherosclerosis
Endocrine	Adrenal suppression Diabetes mellitus Menstrual irregularities
Neurological	Insomnia Depression Euphoria Psychosis
Ocular	Cataracts Glaucoma
Haematological	Leucocytosis
Other	Growth retardation in children and adolescents

be affected; whilst some effects occur primarily at high dosages many occur with low-dose therapy (Saag *et al.* 1994; Committee on Safety of Medicines 1997). Specific guidance on the safe use of corticosteroids has been issued by the Committee on Safety of Medicines (1994, 1998).

Disease severity is an important confounding factor in most studies as traditionally systemic corticosteroid therapy has been reserved for those with more severe disease. However, despite adjusting for these variables, prednisolone use has been correlated with the development of a number of adverse events (e.g. serious infection, fracture and gastrointestinal events) in a dose-dependent manner (Committee on Safety of Medicines 1997).

Infection remains a concern in patients receiving corticosteroids and the particular problems concerning chickenpox have been highlighted. The issue of osteoporosis should also be considered (Verstraeten *et al.* 1986). While the evidence that low-dose prednisolone causes osteoporosis in RA patients in conflicting, an association with increased fracture risk has been reported (Michel *et al.* 1991; Leight and Fries 1991). It seems prudent, therefore, to monitor bone mineral density in patients at risk.

Prednisolone use has emerged in several studies as a predictor of mortality in RA (Wolfe *et al.* 1994). It is not clear, however, whether the drug is simply acting as a surrogate marker of disease severity or is in itself implicated in the reduced survival rates.

PRACTICAL PRESCRIBING OF SYSTEMIC CORTICOSTEROIDS

- The lowest possible dose of corticosteroids should be used for the shortest possible time.
- Oral corticosteroids are not recommended routinely in RA, as there is no sustained clinical or functional benefit and further studies are needed to assess the effect on X-ray progression.
- Oral corticosteroids should be withdrawn slowly to avoid rebound flare of symptoms as well as hypoadrenalism.
- IM bridge therapy allows control of dose and duration of therapy and may be preferred.
- Patients should be monitored for adverse effects. Inform patients not previously affected of the danger of chickenpox/shingles exposure.
- Counsel patients fully about the benefits and risks of corticosteroid therapy and issue a steroid warning card.

KEY REFERENCES

- Kirwan *et al.* 1995

- Boers 1997

- Saag 1994

- Laan 1999

- Empire Rheumatism Council 1957

REFERENCES

ACR (2002). 2002 Annual Scientific Meeting. New Orleans, LA: American College of Rheumatology.

Adams EM, Yocum DE, Bell CL (1983). Hydroxychloroquine in the treatment of rheumatoid arthritis *Am J Med* **75**:321–6.

Ahern MJ, Harrison W, Hollingsworth P, Bradley J, Laing B, Bayliss C (1991). A randomized double-blind trial of cyclosporin and azathioprine in refractory rheumatoid arthritis. *Aust NZ J Med* **21**:844–9.

Ahlmen M, Ahlmen J, Svalander C, Bucht H (1987). Cycotoxic drug treatment of reactive amyloidosis in rheumatoid arthritis with special reference to renal insufficiency. *Clin Rheumatol* **6**:27–38.

American College of Rheumatology Ad Hoc Committee on Clinical Guidelines (1996). Guidelines for monitoring drug therapy in rheumatoid arthritis. *Arthritis Rheum* **39**:723–31.

Amos RS, Pullar T, Bax DE, Situnayake D, Capell HA, McConkey (1986). Sulphasalazine for rheumatoid arthritis: toxicity in 774 patients monitored for 1 to 11 years. *Br Med J* **293**:420–3.

Andersen PA, West SG, O'Dell JR *et al.* (1985). Weekly pulse methotrexate in rheumatoid arthritis. Clinical and immunologic effects in a randomized, double-blind study. *Ann Intern Med* **103**:489–96.

Arnold MH, O'Callaghan J, McCredie M, Beller EM, Kelly DE, Brooks PM (1990). Comparative controlled trial of low-dose weekly methotrexate versus azathioprine in rheumatoid arthritis: a 3-year prospective study. *Bri J Rheumatol* **29**:120–5.

Association of the British Pharmaceutical Industry (ABPI) (2000–2001). *Compendium data sheets* **OR** *Datasheet compendium* (ed. G Walker). Datapharm Publications, p. 1205.

Australian Multicentre Clinical Trial Group (1992). Sulfasalazine in early rheumatoid arthritis. *J Rheumatol* **19**:1672–7.

Bailer III, JC (1997). The promise and problems of meta-analysis. *N Engl J Med* **337**:559–61.

Baker GL, Kahl LE, Zee BC *et al.* (1987). Malignancy following treatment of rheumatoid arthritis with cyclophosphamide. *Am J Med* **83**:1–9.

Balint P, Kane D, Hunter J, McInnes IB, Field M, Sturrock R (2002). A comparison of ultrasound-guided with convention joint aspiration in rheumatoid practice—a pilot study. *Rheumatology* (Abst Suppl):118.

Bathon J, Martin R, Fleischmann R *et al.* (2000) A comparison of etanercept and methotrexate in patients with early rheumatoid arthritis. *N Engl J Med* **343**:1586–93.

Beecher HK (1959). *Measurement of subjective responses*. New York: Oxford University Press.

Bellamy N, Buchanan WW, Goldsmith CH, Campbell J, Stitt L (1988). Validation study of WOMAC: A health status instrument for measuring clinically important patient relevant outcomes to anti-rheumatic drug therapy in patients with osteoarthritis of the hip or knee. *J Rheumatol* **15**:1833–40.

Bendix G, Bjelle A (1996). A 10 year follow-up of parenteral gold therapy in patients with rheumatoid arthritis. *Ann Rheum Dis* **55**:169–76.

REFERENCES

Berry H, Liyange SP, Durance RA, Barnes CG, Berger LA, Evans SO (1976). Azathioprine and penicillamine in the treatment of rheumatoid arthritis. *Br Med J* **1**:1052–4.

Bird HA (1994). Intra-articular and intralesional therapy. In *Oxford textbook of rheumatology* (eds JH Klippel, PA Nieppe). St Louis MO: Mosby, Ch 16, pp.16.1–16.6

Bird HA, Le Gallez P, Dixon JS Surrall KE Cole DS *et al.* (1984). A single blind comparative study of auranofin and hydroxychloroquine in patients with rheumatoid arthritis. *Clin Rheumatol* **3**(Suppl):57–66.

Black AJ, McLeod HL, Capell HA *et al.* (1998). Thiopurine methyltransferase genotype predicts therapy-limiting severe toxicity from azathioprine. *Ann Intern Med* **129**:716–18.

Blackburn WD, Prupas HM, Silverfield JC, Poiley JE *et al.* (1995). Tenidap in rheumatoid arthritis. A 24-week double-blind comparison with hydroxychloroquinine-plus-piroxicam and piroxicam alone. *Arthritis Rheum* **38**:1447–56.

Bluhm GB, Sharp JT, Tilley BC *et al.* (1997). Radiographic results from the Minocycline in Rheumatoid Arthritis (MIRA) Trial. *J Rheumatol* **24**:1295–302.

Blyth T, Hunter J, Stirling A (1994). Pain relief in the rheumatoid knee after steroid injection. A single-blind comparison of hydrocortisone succinate and triamcinolone acetonide or hexacetonide. *Br J Rheumatol* **44**:461–3.

Boers M (1999). The case for corticosteroids in the treatment of early rheumatoid arthritis. *Br J Rheumatol* **38**:95–7.

Boers M (2001). NSAIDs and selective COX-2 inhibitors: competition between gastro-protection and cardioprotection. *Lancet* **357**:1222–3.

Boers M, Verhoeven AC, Markusse HM *et al.* (1997). Randomized comparison of combined step-down prednisolone, methotrexate and sulphasalazine with sulphasalazine alone in early rheumatoid arthritis. *Lancet* **350**:309–18.

Bombardier C, Ware J, Russell IJ *et al.* (1986). Auranofin therapy and quality of life in patients with rheumatoid arthritis. Results of a multicenter trial. *Am J Med* **81**:565–78.

Bombardier C, Laine L, Reicin A *et al.* (2000). Comparison of upper gastrointestinal toxicity of rofecoxib and naproxen in patients with rheumatoid arthritis (VIGOR). *N Engl J Med* **343**:1520–8.

Borg G, Allander E, Lund B *et al.* (1988). Auranofin improves outcome in early rheumatoid arthritis. Results from a 2 year, double blind, placebo controlled study. *J Rheumatol* **15**:1747–54.

Borg G, Allander E, Berg E *et al.* (1991). Auranofin treatment in early RA may postpone early retirement. Results from a 2-year, double blind trial. *J Rheumatol* **18**:1015–20.

Braun J, Sieper J (2002). Therapy of ankylosing spondylitis and other spondyloarthritides: established medical treatment, anti-TNF-α therapy and other novel approaches. *Arthritis Res* **4**:307–21.

Bresnihan B, Alvaro-Gracia JM, Cobby M *et al.* (1998). Treatment of rheumatoid arthritis with recombinant human interleukin-1 receptor antagonist. *Arthritis Rheum* **41**(12):2196–204.

British National Formulary (2002a). **42**:484.

British National Formulary (2002b). **43**:486–7.

Brown GJE, Yeomans ND (1999). Prevention of the gastrointestinal adverse effects of non-steroidal anti-inflammatory drugs: the role of proton pump inhibitors. *Drug Safety* **21**:503–12.

Brun J, Jones R (2001). Non-steroidal anti-inflammatory drug-associated dyspepsia: the scale of the problem. *Am J Med* **110**:12S–13S.

Buchanan WW, Kean WF (1987). William Heberden the Elder (1710–1801). The complete physician and sometime rheumatologist. *Clin Pharmacol* **6**:251–63.

Bunch TW, O'Duffy JD, Tompkins RB, O'Fallon WM (1984). Controlled trial of hydroxychloroquine and D-penicillamine singly and in combination in the treatment of rheumatoid arthritis. *Arthritis Rheum* **27**:267–76.

Cade R, Stein G, Pickering M, Schlein E, Spooner G (1976). Low dose, long-term treatment of rheumatoid arthritis with azathioprine. *South Med J* **69**:388–92.

Caldwell JR, Furst D (1991). The efficacy and safety of low-dose corticosteroids for rheumatoid arthritis. *Semin Arth Rheum* **21**:1–11.

Canadian Consensus Conference on Hydroxychloroquine (2000). *J Rheumatology* **27**:2919–21.

Cannon GW, Jackson CG, Samuelson CO Jr, Ward JR, Williams HJ, Clegg DO (1985). Chlorambucil therapy in rheumatoid arthritis: clinical experience with 28 patients and literature review. *Semin Arth Rheum* **15**:106–18.

Capell HA, Lewis D, Carey J (1986). A three year follow up of patients allocated to placebo, or oral or injectable gold therapy for rheumatoid arthritis. *Ann Rheum Dis* **45**:705–11.

Capell HA, Marabani M, Madhok R, Torley H, Hunter JA (1990). Degree and extent of response to sulphasalazine or penicillamine therapy for rheumatoid arthritis: Results from a routine clinical environment over a two year period. *Quart J Med* **75**:335–44.

Capell HA, Maiden N, Madhok R, Hampson R, Thomson EA (1998). Intention-to-treat analysis of 200 patients with rheumatoid arthritis 12 years after random allocation to either sulfasalazine or penicillamine. *J Rheumatol* **25**:1880–6.

Carette S, Calin A, McCafferty JP, Wallin BA (1989). A double blind placebo-controlled study of auranofin in patients with rheumatoid arthritis. *Arthritis Rheum* **32**:158–65.

Carmichael SJ, Beal J, Day RO, Tett SE (2002). Combination therapy with methotrexate and hydroxychloroquine for rheumatoid arthritis increases exposure to methotrexate. *J Rheumatol* **29**:1077–83.

Chakravarty K, Pharoah PDP, Scott DGI (1994). A randomized controlled study of post-injection rest following intra-articular steroid therapy for knee synovitis. *Br J Rheumatol* **33**:464–8.

Chan KBY, Man-Son-Hing M, Molnar FJ, Laupaces A (2001). How well is the clinical importance of study results reported? An assessment of randomized controlled trials. *Canad Med Assoc J* **165**:1197–202.

Chrubasik S, Eisenberg E, Balan E, Weinberger T, Luzzati R, Conradt C (2000). Treatment of low back pain exacerbations with willow bark extract: A randomized double-blind study. *Am J Med* **109**:9–14.

Ciconelli RM, Ferraz MB, Visioni RA, Oliveira LM, Atra E (1996). A randomized double-blind controlled trial of sulphasalazine combined with pulses of methylprednisolone or placebo in the treatment of rheumatoid arthritis. *Br J Rheumatol* **35**:150–4.

Clark P, Casas E, Tugwell P *et al.* (1993) Hydroxychloroquine compared with placebo in rheumatoid arthritis. *Ann Intern Med* **119**:1067–71.

Clarke M, Chalmers I (1998). Discussion sections in reports of controlled trials published in general medical journals: islands in search of continents? *JAMA* **280**:280–2.

Cohen AS, Calkins E (1958). A controlled study if chloroquine as an anti-rheumatic agent. *Arthritis Rheum* **1**:297.

Cohen AS *et al.* (2002). Treatment of rheumatoid arthritis with anakinra, a recombinant human interleukin-1 receptor antagonist in combination with methotrexate. *Arthritis Rheum* **46**:614–24.

Cohen S, Cannon GW, Schiff M *et al.* (2001). Two-year, blinded, randomized, controlled trial of treatment of active rheumatoid arthritis with leflunomide compared with methotrexate. Utilization of Leflunomide in the Treatment of Rheumatoid Arthritis Trial Investigator Group. *Arthritis Rheum* **44**:1984–92.

Comer M, Scott DL, Doyle DV, Huskisson EC, Hopkins A (1995). Are slow-acting anti-rheumatic drugs monitored too often? An audit of current clinical practice. *Br J Rheumatol* **34**:966–70.

Committee on Safety of Medicines (1994). Severe chickenpox associated with systemic corticosteroids. *Curr Probl Pharmacol* **20**:1–2.

Committee on Safety of Medicines (1997). Using long-term corticosteroids safely. *Curr Probl Pharmacol* **23**:4.

Committee on Safety of Medicines (1998). Focus on corticosteroids. *Curr Probl Pharmacol* **24**:5–10.

Conn DL (2002). Resolved: low-dose prednisolone is indicated as a standard treatment in patients with rheumatoid arthritis. *Arth Care Res* **45**:462–7.

Cooperating Clinics Committee of the American Rheumatism Association (1970). A controlled trial of Cyclophosphamide in Rheumatoid Arthritis. *N Engl J Med* **283**:883–9.

Cooperating Clinics Committee of the American Rheumatism Association (1973). A controlled trial of gold salt therapy in rheumatoid arthritis. *Arthritis Rheum* **16**:353.

Corkhill MM, Kirkham BW, Chikanza IC, Gibson T, Panayi GS (1990). Intramuscular depot methylprednisolone induction of chrysotherapy in rheumatoid arthritis: a 24 week randomized controlled trial. *Br J Rheumatol* **29**:274–9.

Criswell LA, Saag KG, Sems KM *et al.* (2002). Moderate-term, low-dose corticosteroids for rheumatoid arthritis (Cochrane Review). *The Cochrane Library*, Issue 1. Oxford: Update Software.

Csuka ME, Carrera GF, McCarty DJ (1986). Treatment of intractable rheumatoid arthritis with combined cyclophosphamide, azathioprine and hydroxychloroquine. *JAMA* **255**: 2315–19.

Currey HLF, Harris J, Mason RM *et al.* (1974). Comparison of azathioprine, and gold in treatment of rheumatoid arthritis. *Br Med J* **3**:763–6.

Data Sheet Ridaura (Tiltab). 1997 Revision

Davis MJ, Dawes PT, Fowler PD, Clarke S, Fisher S, Shadforth MF (1991). Should disease-modifying agents be used in mild rheumatoid arthritis? *Br J Rheumatol* **30**:451–4.

Davis P, Menard H, Thomson J, Harth M, Beaudet F (1985). One year comparison of gold sodium thiomalate and auranofin in the treatment of rheumatoid arthritis. *J Rheumatol* **12**:60–7.

Deeks JJ, Smith LA, Bradley MD (2002). Efficacy, tolerability and upper gastrointestinal safety of celecoxib for treatment of osteoarthritis and rheumatoid arthritis: systematic review of randomized controlled trials. *BMJ* **325**:619–23.

Dennison E, Cooper C (1998). Corticosteroids in rheumatoid arthritis. *BMJ* **316**:789–90.

Dixon A St J, Davis J, Dormandy TL *et al.* (1975). Synthetic (D-) penicillamine in rheumatoid arthritis. *Ann Rheum Dis* **34**:416–21.

Docherty M, Smith R (1999). The case for structuring the discussion of scientific papers. *BMJ* **318**:1224–5.

Doherty M, Hazleman BL, Hutton CW, Maddison PJ, Perry JD (1992). *Rheumatology examination and injection techniques.* Philadelphia: WB Saunders.

Dougados M, Awada H, Amor B (1998). Cyclosporin in rheumatoid arthritis: a double blind, placebo controlled study in 52 patients. *Ann Rheum Dis* **47**:127–33.

Dougados M, Combe B, Cantagrel A *et al.* (1999). Combination therapy in early rheumatoid arthritis: a randomized controlled double blind 52 week clinical trial of sulphasalazine and methotrexate compared with the single components. *Ann Rheum Dis* **58**:220–5.

Downie RS, Macnaughton J (eds) (2000). *Clinical judgement evidence in practice.* Oxford, UK: Oxford University Press.

Drosos AA, Voulgari PV, Katsaraki A, Zikou AK (2000). Influence of cyclosporin A on radiological progression in early rheumatoid arthritis patients: a 42-month prospective study. *Rheumatol Int* **19**:113–18.

Dwosh IL, Stein HB, Urowitz MB, Smythe HA, Hunter T, Ogryzlo MA (1977). Azathioprine in early rheumatoid arthritis. Comparison with gold and chloroquine. *Arthritis Rheum* **20**:685–92.

Edwards J, Hannah B, Brailsford-Atkinson K, Price T, Sheeran T, Mulherin D (2002). Intra-articular and soft tissue injections: assessment of the service provided by nurses. *Ann Rheum Dis* **61**:656–7.

Egger M, Davey-Smith G, Sterne JAC (2001). Uses and abuses of meta-analysis. *Clin Med (JRCPL)* **1**:478–84.

Eisenberg DM, Davis RB, Ettner SL *et al.* (1998). Trends in alternative medicine use in the United States: results of a follow-up national survey. *JAMA* **280**:1589–95.

Emery P, Breedveld FC, Lemmel EM *et al.* (2000). A comparison of the efficacy and safety of leflunomide and methotrexate for the treatment of rheumatoid arthritis. *Rheumatology* **39**:655–65.

Empire Rheumatism Council (1957). Multi-centre controlled trial comparing cortisone acetate and acetyl salicylic acid in the long-term treatment of rheumatoid arthritis. *Ann Rheum Dis* **16**:277–89.

Empire Rheumatism Council (1961). Gold therapy in rheumatoid arthritis: final report of a multi-centre controlled trial. *Ann Rheum Dis* **20**:315–34.

Ernst E (1998). Harmless herbs? A review of the recent literature. *Am J Med* **104**:170–87.

Esdaile JM and The HERA Study Group (1995). A randomized trial of hydroxychloroquine in early rheumatoid arthritis: the HERA study. *Am J Med* **98**:156.

Faarvang KL, Egsmose C, Kryger P, Podenphant J, Ingeman-Neilsen M, Hansen TM (1993). Hydroxychloroquine and sulphasalazine alone and in combination in rheumatoid arthritis: a randomized double blind trial. *Ann Rheum Dis* **52**:711–15.

Felix-Davies DD, Stewart AM, Wilkinson AM, Bateman JR, Delamere JP (1983). A 12-month comparative trial of auranofin and D-penicillamine in rheumatoid arthritis. *Am J Med* **75**(Suppl.):138–41.

Felson DT, Anderson JJ, Meenan RF (1990). The comparative efficacy and toxicity of second-line agents in rheumatoid arthritis. Results of two meta-analyses. *Arthritis Rheum* **33**:1449–61.

Felson DT, Anderson JJ, Meenan RF (1992). Use of short-term efficacy/toxicity tradeoffs to select second-line drugs in rheumatoid arthritis: a meta-analysis of published clinical trials. *Arthritis Rheum* **35**:1117–25

Felson DT, Anderson JJ, Meenan RF (1994). The efficacy and toxicity of combination therapy in rheumatoid arthritis. A meta-analysis. *Arthritis Rheum* **37**:1487–91.

Fielder A, Grahjam E, Jones S, Silman A, Tullo A (1998). Royal College of Ophthalmologists Guidelines: ocular toxicity and hydroxychloroquine. *Eye* **12**:907–9.

Finbloom DS Silver K, Newsom DA, Gunkel R (1985). Comparison of Hydroxychloroquine and chloroquine use and development of retinal toxicity. *J Rheumatol* **12:**692–4.

Fitzgerald GA, Patrone C (2001). The coxibs, selective inhibitors of cyclo-oxygenase-2. *N Engl J Med* **345**:433–42.

Fitzgerald O, Hanly J, Callan A, McDonald K, Molony J, Bresnihan B (1985). Effects of joint lavage on knee synovitis in rheumatoid arthritis. *Br J Rheumatol* **24**:6–10.

Forestier JM (1929). *Bulletin et Mémoires de la Societé Médicale de Hopitaux de Paris* **53**:323.

Forre O (1994). Radiologic evidence of disease modification in rheumatoid arthritis patients treated with cyclosporine. Results of a 48 week multicenter study comparing low-dose cyclosporine with placebo. Norwegian Arthritis Study Group. *Arthritis Rheum* **37**:1506–12.

Forre O, Bjerkhoel F, Salvesen CF *et al.* (1987). An open, controlled, randomized comparison of cyclosporine and azathioprine in the treatment of rheumatoid arthritis: a preliminary report. *Arthritis Rheum* **30**:88–92.

Fraser TN (1945). Gold treatment in rheumatoid arthritis. *Ann Rheum Dis* **4**:1–75.

Furst DE (1990). Rational use of disease-modifying antirheumatic drugs. *Drugs* **39**:19–37.

Furst DE, Lindsley H, Baethge B *et al.* (1999). Dose-loading with hydroxychloroquine improves the rate of response in early, active rheumatoid arthritis. *Arthritis Rheum* **42**:357–65.

Gaffney K, Scott DGI (1998). Azathioprine and cyclophosphamide in the treatment of rheumatoid arthritis. *Br J Rheumatol* **37**:824–36.

Genovese MC, Bathon JM, Martin RW *et al.* (2002). Etanercept versus methotrexate in patients with early rheumatoid arthritis: two-year radiographic and clinical outcomes. *Arthritis Rheum* **46**:1443–50.

Gerards AH, Landewé RB, Prins APA *et al.* (2003). Cyclosporin A monotherapy versus cyclosporin A and methotrexate combination therapy in patients with early rheumatoid arthritis: a double blind randomised placebo controlled trial. *Ann Rheum Dis* **62**:291–6.

Giannini EH. Cassidy JT. Brewer EJ *et al.* (1993) Comparative efficacy and safety of advanced drug therapy in children with juvenile rheumatoid arthritis. *Semin Arthritis Rheum* **23**:34–46.

Gibson T, Huskissson EC, Wojtulewski JA *et al.* (1976) Evidence that D-penicillamine alters the course of rheumatoid arthritis. *Rheumatol Rehabil* **15**:211–15.

Glennas A, Kvien TK, Andrup O *et al.* (1997). Auranofin is safe and superior to placebo in elderly-onset rheumatoid arthritis. *Br J Rheumatol* **36**:870–7.

Gofton JP, O'Brien WM, Hurley KN, Scheffler BJ (1984). Radiographic evaluation of erosion in in rheumatoid arthritis; double blind study of auranofin vs placebo. *J Rheumatol* **11**:768–71.

Goldman JA, Myerson G (1991). Chinese herbal medicine: camouflaged prescription anti-inflammatory drugs, corticosteroids and lead. *Arthritis Rheum* **34**:1207.

Gorman JD, Sack KE, Davis JC Jr (2002). Treatment of ankylosing spondylitis by inhibition of tumor necrosis factor alpha. *N Engl J Med* **346**(18):1349–56.

Gotzsche PC, Podenphant I, Olesen M, Halberg P (1992). Meta-analysis of second-line anti-rheumatic drugs: Sample size bias and uncertain benefit. *J Clin Epidemiol* **45**:587–94.

Gotzsche PC, Johansen HK (1998). Meta-analysis of short term low dose prednisolone versus placebo and non-steroidal anti-inflammatory drugs in rheumatoid arthritis. *BMJ* **316**:811–18.

Gould SJ (1996). Death and horses: two cases for the primary of variation. In *Full house. The spread of excellence from Plato to Darwin*. New York: Harmony Books, pp.43–73.

Grassi W, Lamanna G, Farina A, Cervini C (1999). Synovitis of small joints: a sonographic guided diagnostic approach. *Ann Rheum Dis* **58**:595–7.

Grierson DJ (1997). Hydroxychloroquine and visual screening in a rheumatology outpatient clinic. *Ann Rev Rheumatol* **56**:188–90.

Guyatt G, Heything A, Jaeschke R *et al.* (1990). N-of-1. Randomized trials for investigating new drugs. *Controlled Clin Trials* **11**:88–100.

Haagsma C, van Riel P, de Jong A, van de Putte L (1997). Combination of sulphasalazine and methotrexate versus the single components in early RA: a randomized controlled double blind 52 week clinical trial. *Br J Rheumatol* **36**:1082–8.

Halberg P, Bentzon MW, Crohn O *et al.* (1984). Double-blind trial of levamisole, penicillamine and azathioprine in rheumatoid arthritis: clinical, biochemical, radiographic and scintigraphic studies. *Danish Med Bull* **31**:403–9.

Hall AG, Tilby MJ (1992). Mechanisms of action of, and modes of resistance to, alkylating agents used in the treatment of haematological malignancies. *Blood Reviews* **6**:163–73.

Hamdy H, McKendry RJR, Mierins E, Liver JA (1987). Low dose methotrexate compared with azathioprine in the treatment of rheumatoid arthritis: a twenty-four week controlled clinical trial. *Arthritis Rheum* **30**:361–8.

Hamilton EBD, Scott JT (1962). Hydroxychloroquine sulphate in treatment of rheumatoid arthritis. *Arthritis Rheum* **5**:502.

Hamilton J, McInnes IB, Thomson EA *et al.* (2001). Comparative study of intramuscular gold and methotrexate in a rheumatoid arthritis population from a socially deprived area. *Ann Rheum Dis* **60**:566–72.

Hannonen P, Möttönen T, Hakola M, Oka M *et al.* (1993). Sulfasalazine in early rheumatoid arthritis. A 48-week double-blind, prospective, placebo-controlled study. *Arthritis Rheum* **36**:1501–9.

Hansen TM, Dickmeiss E, Jans H, Hansen TI, Ingeman-Neilsen M, Lorenzen IB (1987). Combination of methylprednisolone pulse therapy and remission inducing drugs in rheumatoid arthritis. *Ann Rheum Dis* **46**:290–5.

Hansen TM, Kryger P, Elling H *et al.* (1990). Double blind placebo controlled trial of pulse treatment withmethylprednisolone combined with disease modifying drugs in rheumatoid arthritis. *BMJ* **301**:268–70.

Harth M, Davis P, Thomson JM, Menard H, Beaudet F (1987). Comparison between sodium aurothiomalate and auranofin in rheumatoid arthritis. Results of a two-year open randomized study. *Scand J Rheumatol* **16**:177–84.

Health Technology Board: www.htbs.co.uk

Heberden W (1994). ANTIΘHPIAKA. An essay on mithridatium and therica. In: *An introduction to the study of physic*. L Crummer, 1929, reprinted by the Classics of Medicine Library, Division of Gryphon Library, New York, pp.20–2.

Hench PS, Kendall EC, Slocumb CH, Polley HF (1949). The effect of a hormone of the adrenal cortex (17-hydroxy-11-dehydrocortisone: compound E) and of pituitary adrenocorticotrophic hormone on rheumatoid arthritis. *Proc Staff Meet Mayo Clin* **24**:181–97.

Henry D, Lim LL-Y, Garcia Rodriguez LA *et al.* (1996). Variability in risk of gastrointestinal complications with individual non-steroidal anti-inflammatory drugs: results of a collaborative meta-analysis. *BMJ* 3**12**:1563–6.

HERA Study Group (1995). A randomized trial of hydroxychloroquine in early rheumatoid arthritis: the HERA study. *Am J Med* **98**:156–68.

Hernandes-Diaz S, Garcia Rodriguez LA (2000). Association between non-steroidal anti-inflammatory drugs and upper gastrointestinal tract bleeding/perforation. *Arch Intern Med* **160**:2093–9.

Hickling P, Jacoby RK, Kirwan JR (1998). Joint destruction after glucocorticosteroids are withdrawn in early rheumatoid arthritis. *Br J Rheumatol* **37**:930–6.

Hochberg MC (1986) Auranofin or D-penicillamine in the treatment of rheumatoid arthritis. *Ann Intern Med* **105**:528–35.

Hunter T, Urorwitz MB, Gordon DA, Smythe HA, Ogryzlo MA (1975). Azathioprine in rheumatoid arthritis. A long-term follow-up study. *Arthritis Rheum* **18**:15–20.

Jeon KI, Jeong JY, Jue DM (2000). Thio-reactive metal compounds inhibits NF-kappa B activation by blocking I kappa B kinase. *J Immunol* **164**:5981–9.

Jessop JD, O'Sullivan MM, Lewis PA *et al.* (1998). A long term five year randomized controlled trial of hydroxychloroquine, sodium aurothiomalate, auranofin and penicillamine in the treatment of patients with rheumatoid arthritis. *Br J Rheum* **37**:992–1002.

Jeurissen M, Boerbooms A, van de Putte L *et al.* (1991a). Methotrexate versus azathioprine in the treatment of rheumatoid arthritis. *Arthritis Rheum* **34**:961–72.

Jeurissen ME, Boerbooms AM, van de Putte LB *et al.* (1991b). Influence of methotrexate and azathioprine on radiologic progression in rheumatoid arthritis. A randomized, double-blind study. *Ann Intern Med* **114**:999–1004.

Jiang Y, Genant HK, Watt I *et al.* (2000). A multicenter, double-blind, dose-ranging, randomized, placebo-controlled study of recombinant human interleukin-1 receptor antagonist in patients with rheumatoid arthritis: radiologic progression and correlation of Genant and Larsen scores. *Arthritis Rheum* **43**:1001–19.

Joint Committee of the Medical Research Council and Nuffield Foundation (1959). A comparison of prednisolone with aspirin or other analgesics in the treatment of rheumatoid arthritis. *Ann Rheum Dis* **18**:173–88.

Joint Committee of the Medical Research Council and Nuffield Foundation (1960). A comparison of prednisolone with aspirin or other analgesics in the treatment of rheumatoid arthritis. *Ann Rheum Dis* **19**:331–7.

Jones A, Regan M, Ledingham J, Pattrick M, Manhire A, Doherty M (1993). Importance of placement of intra-articular steroid injections. *BMJ* **307**:1329–30.

Jones E, Jones JV, Woodbury JFL (1991). Response to sulfasalazine in rheumatoid arthritis: life table analysis of a 5-year followup. *J Rheumatol* **18**:195–8.

Jones G, Crotty M, Brooks P *et al.* (1959). Psoriatic arthritis: a quantitative overview of therapeutic options. *Br J Rheumatol* **36**:95–9.

Joyce CRB (1994). Placebo and complementary medicine. *Lancet* **344**:1279–81.

Juni P, Rutjes AWS, Dieppe PA (2002). Are selective COX 2 inhibitors superior to traditional non-steroidal anti-inflammatory drugs? Adequate analysis of the CLASS trial indicates that this may not be the case. *BMJ* **324**:1287–8.

Kahn M, de Seze S (1974). Immunosuppressive agents in rheumatology. Indications, results, and long-term adverse effects. *Ann Med Intern (Paris)* **125**:449–506.

Katz WA, Alexander S, Bland JH *et al.* (1982). The efficacy and safety of auranofin compared to placebo in rheumatoid arthritis. *J Rheumatol* **9**(Suppl):173–8.

Kean WF, Hart L, Buchanan WW (1997). Auranofin. *Br J Rheumatol* **36**:560–72.

Kersley GD, Palin AG (1959). Amodiaquine and hydroxychloroquine in rheumatoid arthritis. *Lancet* **2**:885.

Kerstens PJSM, Boerbooms AMTh, Jeurissen MEC, de Graaf R, Mulder J, van de Putte LBA (2000). Radiological and clinical results of long term treatment of rheumatoid arthritis with methotrexate and azathioprine. *J Rheumatol* **27**:1148–55.

Keysser G, Keysser C, Keysser M (1998). Treatment of refractory rheumatoid arthritis with low-dose cyclophosphamide. Long-term follow-up of 108 patients. *Z Rheumatol* **57**:101–7.

Kinlen LJ, Sheil AGR, Peto R, Doll R (1979). A collaborative UK-Australian study of cancer in patients treated with immunosuppressive drugs. *Br Med J* **ii**:1461–4.

Kirwan JR (1995). The effect of glucocorticoids on joint destruction in rheumatoid arthritis. *N Engl J Med* **333**:142–6.

Kloppenburg M, Breedveld FC, Terwiel JP, Mallee C, Dijkmans BA (1994). Minocucline in active rheumatoid arthritis. A double-blind, placebo-controlled trial. *Arthritis Rheum* **37**:629–36.

Krogstad D, Schlesinger M (1987) Acid vesical function, intracellular pathogens, and the action of chloroquine against plasmodium phalsiparum. *N Engl J Med* **317**:542–9.

Kruger K, Schattenkirchner M (1994). Comparison of cyclosporin A and azathioprine in the treatment of rheumatoid arthritis—results of a double-blind multicentre study. *Clin Rheumatol* **13**(2):248–55.

Kvien TK, Zeidler HK, Hannonen P *et al.* (2002). Long term efficacy and safety of cyclosporin versus parenteral gold in early rheumatoid arthritis: a three year study of radiographic progression, renal function, and arterial hypertension. *Ann Rheum Dis* **61**:511–16.

La Corte R, Caselli M, Castellino G *et al.* (1999). Prophylaxis and treatment of NSAID-induced gastroduodenal disorders. *Drug Safety* **20**(6):527–43.

Laan RFJM, Jansen TLThA, van Riel PLCM (1999). Glucocorticoids in the management of rheumatoid arthritis. *Rheumatol* **38**:6–12.

Larsen A, Kvien TK, Schattenkirchner M *et al.* (2001). Slowing of disease progression in rheumatoid arthritis patients during long-term treatment with leflunomide or sulphasalazine. *Scand J Rheumatol* **30**:135–42.

Leake J (1995). Thousands fight for steroid justice. *Sunday Times* August 27.

Lee P, Webb J, Anderson JA, Buchanan WW (1973). A method for assessing the therapeutic potential of anti-inflammatory anti-rheumatic drugs in rheumatoid arthritis. *Brit Med J* **2**:685–8.

Lehtinen K, Isomäki H (1991). Intramuscular gold therapy is associated with long survival in patients with rheumatoid arthritis. *J Rheumatol* **18**:524–9.

Leigh JP, Fries JF (1991). Mortality predictors among 263 patients with rheumatoid arthritis. *J Rheumatol* **18**:1307–12.

Levy J, Paulus HE, Bangert R (1975). Comparison of azathioprine and cyclophosphamide in the treatment of rheumatoid arthritis. *Arthritis Rheum* **18**:412–13.

Levy M, Buskila D, Gladman DD, Urowitz MU, Koren G (1991). Pregnancy outcome following first trimester exposure to chloroquine. *Am J Perinatology* **8**:174–8.

Levy J, Paulus HE, Sokoloff M, Bangert R, Pearson CM (1972). A double-blind controlled evaluation of azathioprine treatment in rheumatoid arthritis and psoriatic arthritis. *Arthritis Rheum* **15**(1):116–17.

Lewis D, Capell HA (1984). Oral gold; a comparison with placebo and with intramuscular sodium aurothiomalate. *Clin Rheumatol* **3**(Suppl):83–96.

Lidsky MD, Sharp JT, Billings S (1973). Double blind study of cyclophosphamide in rheumatoid arthritis. *Arthritis Rheum* **16**:148–52.

Liebling MR, Leib E, McLaughlin K *et al.* (1981). Pulse methylprednisolone in rheumatoid arthritis. A double-blind cross-over trial. *Ann Intern Med* **94**:21–6.

Lind J (1753). *A treatise of the scurvy.* Edinburgh: Sands, Murray and Cochran.

Lipsky PE, van der Heijde DM, St Clair EW *et al.* (2000). Infliximab and methotrexate in the treatment of rheumatoid arthritis. *N Engl J Med* **343**:1594–602

Lopez-Mendez A, Daniel WW, Reading JC, Ward JR, Alarcon GS (1993). Radiographic assessment of disease progression in rheumatoid arthritis patients enrolled in the cooperative systematic studies of the rheumatic diseases programme randomized clinical trial of methotrexate, auranofin or a combination of the two. *Arthritis Rheum* **36**:1364–9.

Louis PCA (1835). *Recherches sur les effets de la saignée dans quelques maladies inflammatoires, et sur l'action de l'émétique et des vésicatoines dans la pneumonie.* Paris: DB Ballière.

Lovell DJ, Giannini EH, Reiff A *et al.* (2000). Etanercept in children with polyarticular juvenile rheumatoid arthritis. *N Engl J Med* **342:**763–9

Maetzel A, Wond A, Strand V, Tugwell P, Wells G, Bombardier C (2000). Meta-analysis of treatment termination rates among rheumatoid arthritis patients receiving disease-modifying anti-rheumatic drugs. *Rheumatology* **39**:975–81.

Maini RN, Breedveld FC, Kalden J *et al.* (1998). Therapeutic efficacy of multiple intravenous infusions of anti-TNF monoclonal antibody combined with low dose weekly methotrexate in rheumatoid arthritis. *Arthritis Rheum* **41**:1552–63.

Maini RN, St Clair EW, Breedveld FC *et al.* (1999). Infliximab (anti-tumour necrosis factor monoclonal antibody) versus placebo in rheumatoid arthritis patients receiving concomitant methotrexate: a randomized phase III trial. *Lancet* **354**:1932–9.

Mainland D, Sutcliffe MI (1962) Hydroxychloroquine sulphate in rheumatoid arthritis: a six month review *Bull Rheum Dis* **13**:287.

Mamdani M, Rochon PA, Juurlink DN *et al.* (2002). Observational study of upper gastrointestinal haemorrhage in elderly patients given selective cyclo-oxygenase-2 inhibitors or conventional non-steroidal anti-inflammatory drugs. *BMJ* **325**:624–7.

Marchesoni A, Battafarano N, Arreghini M *et al.* (2002). Step-down approach using either cyclosporin A or methotrexate as maintenance therapy in early rheumatoid arthritis. *Arthritis Rheum* **47**:59–66.

Marks JS, Power BJ (1979). Is chloroquine obsolete in the treatment of rheumatic disease? *Lancet* **1**:371–3.

Martindale. *The complete drug reference*, 32 edn (ed. K Parfitt). London: Pharmaceutical Press, pp.19–20.

Mason M, Currey HLF, Barnes CG, Dunne JF, Hazleman BL, Strickland ID (1969). Azathioprine in rheumatoid arthritis. *Brit Med J* **1**:420–2.

Mavrikakis M, Papazoglou S, Sfikakis PP, Vaiopoulos G, Rougas K (1996). Retinal toxicity in long term hydroxychloroquine treatment. *Ann Rheum Dis* **55**:187–9.

Max MB, Schafer SC, Culnane J *et al.* (1988). Association of pain relief with drug side-effects in post-herpetic neuralgia. *Clin Pharmacol Ther* **43**:363–71.

McConkey B, Amos RS, Durham S, Forster PJG, Hubball S, Walsh L (1980). Sulphasalazine in rheumatoid arthritis. *Brit Med J* **i**:442–4.

McEntegart A, Porter D, Capell HA, Thomson EA (1996). Sulfasalazine has a better efficacy/toxicity profile then auranofin—evidence from a 5 year prospective, randomized trial. *J Rheumatol* **23**:1887–90.

Menninger H, Herborn G, Sander O *et al.* (1988). A 36 month comparative trial of methotrexate and gold sodium thiomalate in the treatment of early active and erosive rheumatoid arthritis. *Br J Rheumatol* **37**:1060–8.

Michel BA, Bloch DA, Fries JF (1991). Predictors of fractures in early rheumatoid arthritis. *J Rheumatol* **18**:804–8.

Morassut P, Goldstein R, Cyr M, Karsh J, McKendry RJR (1989). Gold sodium thiomalate compared to low dose methotrexate in the treatment of rheumatoid arthritis—a randomized, double blind 26 week trial. *J Rheumatol* **16**:302–6.

Moreland LW, Baumgartner SW, Schiff MH *et al.* (1997). Treatment of rheumatoid arthritis with a recombinant human tumor necrosis factor receptor (p75)-Fc fusion protein. *N Engl J Med* **337**(3):141–7.

Moreland LW, Schiff MH, Baumgartner SW *et al.* (1999). Etanercept therapy in rheumatoid arthritis. A randomized, controlled trial. *Ann Intern Med* **130**(6):478–86.

Morgan S, Baggott J, Vaughn W *et al.* (1990). The effect of folic acid supplementation on the toxicity of low dose methotrexate in patients with rheumatoid arthritis. *Arthritis Rheum* **33**:9–18.

Morrison E, Capell H (1999). Corticosteroids in rheumatoid arthritis—the case against. *Br J Rheumatol* **38**:97–100.

Möttönen T, Hannonen P, Leirisalo-Repo M *et al.* (1999). Comparison of combination therapy with single-drug therapy in early rheumatoid arthritis: a randomised trial. *Lancet* **353**: 1568–73.

Multi-centre Trial Group (1973). Controlled trial of D(-) penicillamine in severe rheumatoid arthritis. *Lancet* **1**:275–80.

Munro R, Capell H (1997). Disease modifying drug series: penicillamine. *Brit J Rheumatol* **36**:104–9.

Munro R, Morrison E, McDonald AG, Hunter JA, Madhok R, Capell HA (1997). Effect of disease modifying agents I on the lipid profiles of patients with rheumatoid arthritis. *Ann Rheum Dis* **56**:374–7.

Munro R, Hampson R, McEntegart A, Thomson EA, Madhok R, Capell HA (1998). Improved functional outcome in patients with early rheumatoid arthritis treated with intramuscular gold: results of a five year prospective study. *Ann Rheum Dis* **57**:88–93.

Munster T, Gibbs JP, Shen D *et al.* (2002). Hydroxychloroquine concentration-response relationships in patients with rheumatoid arthritis. *Arthritis Rheum* **46**:1460–9.

REFERENCES

National Institute for Clinical Excellence (NICE) Appraisal Team (2000 & 2001). *The clinical effectiveness and cost effectiveness of celecoxib, rofecoxib, meloxicam and etodolac (COX-2 inhibitors) for rheumatoid arthritis and osteoarthritis.* November 2000. Plus Assessment Report addendum prepared by the NICE Appraisals Team, February 2001.

National Institute for Clinical Excellence (NICE) (2001). Guidance on the use of cyclo-oxygenase (Cox) II selective inhibitors, celecoxib, rofecoxib, meloxicam and etodolac for osteoarthritis and rheumatoid arthritis. *Technology Appraisal Guidance* No. 27, July.

Neumann V, Grindulis K, Hubbal S, McConkey B, Wright V (1983). Comparison between penicillamine and sulphasalazine in rheumatoid arthritis. *Br Med J* **287**:1099–102.

Nordle O, Brantmark R (1977). A self-adjusting randomization plan for allocating of patients into two treatment groups. *Clin Pharmacol Ther* **22**:825–30.

Nuver-Zwart IH, van Riel PLCM, van de Putte LBA, Gribnau FWJ (1989). A double blind comparative study of sulphasalazine and hydroxychloroquine in rheumatoid arthritis: evidence of an earlier effect of sulphasalazine. *Ann Rheum Dis* **48**:389–95.

O'Brien WM, Bagby GF (1985). Rare adverse reactions to non-steroidal anti-inflammatory drugs. *J Rheum* **12**:13–20. 2. 2: 347–53. 3. 562–7. 4. 785–90.

O'Dell JR, Haire CE, Erikson N *et al.* (1996). Treatment of rheumatoid arthritis with methotrexate alone, sulfasalazine and hydroxychloroquine or a combination of all three medications. *N Engl J Med* **334**:1287–91.

O'Dell JR, Haire CE, Palmer W *et al.* (1997). Treatment of early rheumatoid arthritis with minocycline or placebo: results of a randomized, double-blind, placebo-controlled trial. *Arthritis Rheum* **40**(5):842–8.

O'Dell JR, Blakely KW, Mallek JA *et al.* (2001). Treatment of early seropositive rheumatoid arthritis: a two-year, double-blind comparison of minocycline and hydroxychloroquine. *Arthritis Rheum* **44**(10):2235–41.

O'Dell JR, Leff R, Paulsen G *et al.* (2002) Treatment of rheumatoid arthritis with methotrexate and hydroxychloroquine, methotrexate and sulfasalazine or a combination of the three medications. *Arthritis Rheum* **46**:1164–70.

Ostensen M (2001). Rheumatological disorders. *Best Pract Res Clin Obstet Gynecol* **15**:953–69.

Parke AL (1988). Antimalarial drugs, systemic lupus erythematosus and pregnancy. *J Rheumatol* **15**:607–10.

Paulus HE, Williams HJ, Ward JR *et al.* (1984). Azathioprine versus d-penicillamine in rheumatoid arthritis patients who have been treated unsuccessfully with gold. *Arthritis Rheum* **27**:721–7.

Pavelka K, Pavelka K, Peliskova Z, Vacha J, Trnavsky K (1989). Hydroxychloroquine sulphate in the treatment of rheumatoid arthritis: a double blind comparison of two dose regimes. *Ann Rheum Dis* **48**:542–6.

Peterson WL (1991). *Helicobacter pylori* and peptic ulcer disease. *N Engl J Med* 1991; **324**:1043–8.

Petri M, Lakatta C, Magder L, Goldman D (1994). Effect of prednisone and hydroxychloroquine on coronary artery disease risk factors in systemic lupus erythematosus: a longitudinal data analysis. *Am J Med* **96:**254–9.

Pinals R, Kaplan SB, Lawson JG, Hepburn B (1986). Sulfasalazine in rheumatoid arthritis. A double-blind, placebo-controlled trial. *Arthritis Rheum* 1986; **29**(12):1427–34.

Porter D, Madhok R, Hunter JA, Capell HA (1992). Prospective trial comparing the use of sulphasalazine and auranofin as second line drugs in patients with rheumatoid arthritis. *Ann Rheum Dis* **51**:461–4.

Porter DR, Capell HA, Hunter J (1993). Combination therapy in rheumatoid arthritis—No benefit of addition of hydroxychloroquine to patients with a suboptimal response to intramuscular gold therapy. *J Rheumatol* **20**:645–9.

Porter DR, McInnes I, Hunter J, Capell HA (1994). Outcome of second line therapy in rheumatoid arthritis. *Ann Rheum Dis* **53**:812–15.

Prete PE, Zane J, Krailo M, Bulanowski M (1994). Randomized trial of switching rheumatoid arthritis patients in remission with injectable gold to auranofin. *Clin Rheumatol* **13**:60–9.

Proudman SM, Conaghan PG, Richardson C *et al.* (2000). Treatment of poor-prognosis early rheumatoid arthritis. A randomized study of treatment with methotrexate, cyclsporin A, and intra-articular corticosteroids compared with sulfasalazine alone. *Arthritis Rheum* **43**:180–19.

Pullar T, Hunter JA, Capell HA (1983). Sulphasalazine in rheumatoid arthritis: a double blind comparison of sulphasalazine with placebo and sodium aurothiomalate. *Brit Med J* **287**:1102–4.

Pullar T, Hunter JA, Capell HA (1987). Effect of sulphasalazine on the radiological progression of rheumatoid arthritis. *Ann Rheum Dis* **46**:398–402.

Rau R, Schattenkirchner M, Muller-Fassbender H *et al.* (1990). A three year comparative study of auranofin and gold sodium thiomalate in rheumatoid arthritis. *Clin Rheumatol* **9**:461–74.

Rau R, Herborn G, Karger T *et al.* (1991). A double blind randomized parallel trial of intramuscular methotrexate and gold sodium thiomalate in early erosive rheumatoid arthritis. *J Rheumatol* **18**:328–33.

Rau R, Herborn G, Menniger H, Blechschmidt J (1997). Comparison of intramuscular methotrexate and gold sodium thiomalate in the treatment of early erosive rheumatoid arthritis: 12 month data of a double-blind parallel study of 174 patients. *Br J Rheumatol* **36**:345–52.

Rau R, Herborn G, Menninger H, Sangha O (1998). Progression in early erosive rheumatoid arthritis: 12 month results from a randomized controlled trial comparing methotrexate and gold sodium thiomalate. *Br J Rheumatol* **37**:1220–6.

Rau R, Herborn G, Menninger H, Sangha O (2002). Radiographic outcome after three years of patients with early erosive rheumatoid arthritis treated with intramuscular methotrexate or parenteral gold. Extension of a one-year double-blind study in 174 patients. *Rheumatology (Oxford)* **41**(2):196–204.

Research Sub-Committee of the Empire Rheumatism Council (1960). Gold therapy in rheumatoid arthritis. *Ann Rheum Dis* **19**:95.

Rice-Evans CA, Miller NJ, Bolwell PG *et al.* (1995). The relative antioxidant activities of plant-derived flavonoids. *Free Rad Res* **32**:375–83.

Rinehart RE, Rosenbaum EE, Hopkins CE (1957). Chloroquine therapy in rheumatoid arthritis. *Northwest Medicine* **56**:703.

Rohnert U, Koske D, Schneider W, Elstner EF (1998). Inhibition by salix extracts and phytodolor of copper-catalysed oxidative destructions. *J Biosciences* **53c**:241–9.

Rosner F (1993). Pharmacology and dietetics in the Bible and Talmud. In: *The healing past. Pharmaceuticals in the biblical and rabbinic world* (eds Jacob, W Jacob). Leiden: EJ Brill, pp.1–26.

Rostom A, Wells G, Tugwell P et al. (2002). Prevention of NSAID-induced gastroduodenal ulcers (Cochrane Review). *The Cochrane Library*, Issue 2. Oxford: Update Software.

Saag KG (2001). Resolved: Low-dose glucocorticoids are neither safe nor effective for the long-term treatment of rheumatoid arthritis. *Arth Care Res* **45**:468–71.

Saag KG, Koehnke R, Caldwell JR et al. (1994). Low dose low-term corticosteroid therapy in rheumatoid arthritis: An analysis of serious adverse events. *Am J Med* **96**:115–23.

Sackett DL, Gent M (1979). Controversy in counting and attributing events in clinical trials. *N Engl J Med* **301**:1401–12.

Saff KG, Criswell LA, Sems KM, Nettleman MD, Kolluri S (1996). Low-dose corticostoids in rheumatoid arthritis. A meta-analysis of their moderate-term effectiveness. *Arthritis Rheum* **39**:1818–25.

Salmaron G, Lipksy PE (1983). Immunosuppressive potential of anti-malarials. *Am J Med* **75**(Suppl A):19–24.

Sanders M (2000). A review of controlled clinical trials examining the effects of antimalarial compounds and gold compounds on radiographic progression in rheumatoid arthritis. *J Rheumatol* **27**:523–9.

Scattenkirchner M, Broll H, Kaik B et al. (1988). Auranofin and gold sodium thiomalate in the treatment of rheumatoid arthritis; a one-year, double blind, comparative multicenter study. *Klinische Wochenschrift* **66**:167–74.

Schmid B, Kötter I, Heide L (2001). Pharmacokinetics of salicin after oral administration of a standardised willow bark extract. *Eur J Clin Pharmacol* **57**:387–91.

Scott DL, Smolen JS, Kalden JR et al. (2001). Treatment of active rheumatoid arthritis with leflunomide: two year follow up of a double blind, placebo controlled trial versus sulphasalazine. *Ann Rheum Dis* **60**:913–23.

Scottish Intercollegiate Guidelines Network (SIGN) (2000). *Management of early rheumatoid arthritis*. Edinburgh: SIGN, pp.48.

Seror P, Pluvinage P, Lecoq-Andre F, Benamou P, Attuil G (1999). Frequency of sepsis after local corticosteroid injection (an inquiry on 1,160,000 injections in rheumatological private practice in France). *Rheumatology* **38**:1272–4.

Sharp JT (2000). An overview of radiographic analysis of joint damage in rheumatoid arthritis and its use in meta-analysis. *J Rheumatol* **27**:254–60.

Sharp JT, Strand V, Leung H et al. (2000). Treatment with leflunomide slows radiographic progression of rheumatoid arthritis: results from three randomized controlled trials of leflunomide in patients with active rheumatoid arthritis. Leflunomide Rheumatoid Arthritis Investigators Group. *Arthritis Rheum* **43**(3):495–505.

Shaw D (1998). Risks or remedies? Safety aspects of herbal remedies in the UK. *J Roy Soc Med* **91**:294–6.

Shiokawa Y, Horiuchi Y, Honma M, Kageyama T, Okada T, Azuma T (1977). Clinical evaluation of D-penicillamine by multicentric double-blind comparative study in chronic rheumatoid arthritis. *Arthritis Rheum* **20**:1464–72.

Shiroky J, Neville C, Esdaile J et al. (1993). Low dose methotrexate with leucovirin (folinic acid) in the management of rheumatoid arthritis. *Arthritis Rheum* **36**:795–803.

Sigker JW, Duncan H, Ensign DC (1974). Gold salts in the treatment of rheumatoid arthritis. A double-blind study. *Ann Intern Med* **80**:21–6.

Silman A, Shipley M (1997). Ophthalmological monitoring for hydroxychloroquine toxicity: a scientific review of available data. *Br J Rheumatol* **36**:599–601.

Silman AJ, Petrie J, Hazleman B, Evans SJW (1988). Lymphoproliferative cancer and other malignancy in patients with rheumatoid arthritis treated with azathioprine: a 20 year follow up study. *Ann Rheum Dis* **47**:988–92.

Silverstein F, Graham D, Senior J *et al.* (1995). Misoprostol reduces gastrointestinal complication sin patients with rheumatoid arthritis receiving non-steroidal anti-inflammatory drugs; a randomized, double-blind, placebo-controlled trial. *Ann Intern Med* **123**:241–9.

Silverstein F, Faich G, Goldstein JL *et al.* (2000). Gatrointestinal toxicity with celecoxib vs non-steroidal anti-inflammatory drugs for osteoarthritis and rheumatoid arthritis. The CLASS Study: a randomized controlled trial. *JAMA* **284**:1247–55.

Silverstein F, Simon L, Faich G (2001). Reporting of 6 month vs 12 month data in a clinical trial of celecoxib. *JAMA* **286**:2398–400 (Letter).

Simon R (1986). Confidence intervals for reporting results of clinical trials. *Ann Intern Med* **105**:429–35.

Singh G (1998). Recent considerations in non-steroidal anti-inflammatory drug gastropathy. *Am J Med* **105**(1B):31S–38S.

Singh G, Fries JF, Spitz P, Williams CA (1989). Toxic effects of azathioprine in rheumatoid arthritis. A national post-marketing perspective. *Arthritis Rheum* **32**:837–43.

Situnayake RD, McConkey B (1990). Clinical and laboratory effects of prolonged therapy with sulfasalazine, gold or penicillamine: the effects of disease duration on treatment response. *J Rheumatol* **17**:1268–73.

Smolen JS, Kalden JR, Scott DL *et al.* (1999). Efficacy and safety of leflunomide compared with placebo and sulphasalazine in active rheumatoid arthritis: a double-blind, randomized, multicentre trial. *Lancet* **353**:259–66.

Smyth CJ, Bartholomew BA, Mills DM *et al.* (1975). Cyclophosphamide therapy for rheumatoid arthritis. *Arch Intern Med* **135**:789–93.

Srinivasan A, Amos M, Webley M (1995). The effects of joint washout and steroid injection compared with either joint washout or steroid injection alone in rheumatoid knee effusion. *Br J Rheumatol* **34**:771–3.

Strand V *et al.* for the Leflunomide RA Investigators Group (1999). Treatment of active rheumatoid arthritis with leflunomide compared with placebo and methotrexate. *Arch Intern Med* **159**:2542–50.

Suarez-Almazor ME, Fitzgerald A, Grace M, Russell A (1988). A randomized controlled trial of parenteral methotrexate compared with sodium aurothiomalate (Myochrysine®) in the treatment of rheumatoid arthritis. *J Rheumatol* **15**:753–6.

Suarez-Almazor ME, Belseck E, Shea B, Homik J, Wells G, Tugwell P (2002a). Antimalarials for treating rheumatoid arthritis. In: *The Cochrane Library*, Vol. 2. Oxford.

Suarez-Almazor ME, Belseck E, Schea B, Wells G, Tugwell P (2002b). Cyclophosphamide for treating Rheumatoid Arthritis (Cochrane Review). *The Cochrane Library*, Issue 2. Oxford: Update Software.

Suarez-Almazor ME, Spooner C, Belseck E (2002c). Azathioprine for treating rheumatoid arthritis. Cochrane Musculoskeletal Group. Cochrane Database of Systemic Reviews, Issue 3.

Talar-Williams C, Hijazi YM, Walter McCM *et al.* (1996). Cyclophosphamide induced cystitis and bladder cancer in patients with Wegener's granulomatosis. *Ann Intern Med* **124**: 477–84.

Taves DR (1974). Minimization: a new method of assigning patients to treatment and control groups. *Clin Pharmacol Ther* **15**:443–53.

Tett SE (1993). Clinical pharmacokinetics of slow acting antirheumatic drugs. *Clin Pharmacokinet* **25**:392–407.

Thomas MH, Rothermuch NO, Philps VK, Bergen W, Hendrick SW (1984). Gold vs D-penicillamine double blind and follow-up. *J Rheumatol* **11**:764–7.

Thompson RN, Watts C, Edelman J et al. (1984). A controlled two-centre trial of parenteral methotrexate therapy for refractory rheumatoid arthritis. *J Rheumatol* **11**(6):760–3.

Tilley BC, Alarcon GS, Heyse SP et al. (1995). Minocycline in rheumatoid arthritis. A 48-week, double-blind, placebo-controlled trial. MIRA Trial Group. *Ann Intern Med* **122**(2):81–9.

Townes AS, Sowa JM, Shulman LE (1976). Controlled trial of cyclophosphamide in rheumatoid arthritis. *Arthritis Rheum* **19**:563–73.

Tsakonas E, Fitzgerald AE, Fitzcharles M-A et al. (2000). Consequences of delayed therapy with second-line agents in rheumatoid arthritis: a 3 year follow up on the hydroxychloroquine in early rheumatoid arthritis (HERA) study. *J Rheumatol* **27**:623–9.

Tugwell P, Bennett K, Gent M (1987). Methotrexate in rheumatoid arthritis. *Ann Intern Med* **107**:358–66.

Tugwell P, Bonbardier C, Gent M et al. (1990). Low dose cyclosporin versus placebo in patients with rheumatoid arthritis. *Lancet* **335**:1051–5.

Tugwell P, Pincus T, Yocum D et al. (1995). Combination therapy with cyclosporine and methotrexate in severe rheumatoid arthritis. The Methotrexate-Cyclosporine Combination Study Group. *N Engl J Med* **333**:137–41.

Updated Consensus Statement on tumour necrosis factor blocking agents for the treatment of rheumatoid arthritis and other rheumatic diseases (April 2001). *Ann Rheum Dis* 2001; **60**:iii2–iii5

Urquhart J (2000). Internal medicine in the 21st Century: Controlled drug delivery: Therapeutic and pharmacological aspects. *J Intern Med* **248**:357–76.

Urowitz MB, Gordon DA, Smythe HA, Pruzanski W, Ogryzio MA (1973). Azathioprine in rheumatoid arthritis. A double-blind, cross-over study. *Arthritis Rheum* **16**:411–18.

van der Heijde DM, val Riel PL, Nuver-Zwart IH, Gribnau FW, van de Putte LB (1989). Effects of hydroxychloroquine and sulphasalazine on progression of joint damage in rheumatoid arthritis. *Lancet* **1**:1036–8.

van der Heijde DM, van Riel PLCM, Nuver-Zwart IH, van de Putte LBA (2000). Alternative methods for analysis of radiographic damage in a randomized, double-blind, parallel group clinical trial comparing hydroxychloroquine and sulfasalazine. *J Rheumatol* **27**(2):535–8; discussion 538–9.

van Ede A, Laan R, Rood M et al. (1999). Effect of folic acid and folinic acid supplementation on toxicity and efficacy of methotrexate in rheumatoid arthritis. *Arthritis Rheum* **42**:S380.

van Ede AE, Laan RF, Rood MJ et al. (2001). Effect of folic or folinic acid supplementation on the toxicity and efficacy of methotrexate in rheumatoid arthritis: a forty-eight week, multicenter, randomized, double-blind, placebo-controlled study. *Arthritis Rheum* **44**(7):1515–24.

van Gestel AM, Laan RFJM, Haagsma CJ, Van de Putte LBA, Van Riel PLCM (1995). Oral steroids as bridge therapy in rheumatoid arthritis patients starting with parenteral gold. A randomized double-blind placebo-controlled trial. *Br J Rheumatol* **34**:347–51.

van Jaarsveld CH, Jahangier ZN, Jacobs JW et al. (2000). Toxicity of anti-rheumatic drugs in a randomized clinical trial of early rheumatoid arthritis. *Rheumatol* **39**:1374–82.

van Riel PL, van der Heijde DM, Nuver-Zwart IH et al. (1995a). Radiographic progression in rheumatoid arthritis: results of three comparative trials. *J Rheumatol* **22**:1797–9.

van Riel PLCM, van Gestel AM, van de Putte LBA (1995b). Long-term usage and side-effect profile of sulphasalazine in rheumatoid arthritis. *Br J Rheumatol* **34**(Suppl 2):40–2.

Venning GR (1983a). Identification of adverse reactions to new drugs. 1. What have been the important adverse reactions since thalidomide. *Brit Med J* **286**:199–204.

Venning GR (1983b). Identification of adverse reactions to new drugs. 2. How were 18 important adverse reactions discovered and with what delays? *Brit Med J* **286**:289–93, 365–8.

Venning GR (1983c). Identification of adverse reactions to new drugs. 3. Alerting processes and early warning systems. *Brit Med J* **286**:458–547.

Verstraeten A, Dequeker J (1986). Vertebral and peripheral bone mineral content and fracture incidence in postmenopausal patients with rheumatoid arthritis: effect of low dose corticosteroids. *Ann Rheum Dis* **45**:852–7.

Ward JR, Williams HJ, Boyce *et al.* (1983a). Comparison of aranofin, gold sodium thiomalate, and placebo in the treatment of rheumatoid arthritis. Subsets of responses. *Am J Med* **75**:133–7.

Ward JR, Williams HJ, Egger MJ *et al.* (1983b). Comparison of auranofin, gold sodium thiomalate and placebo in the treatment of rheumatoid arthritis. *Arthritis Rheum* **26**(11):1303–13.

Watson G (1996). *Theriac and mithridatium. A study in therapeutics*. London: The Wellcome Historical Medical Library.

Weinblatt M, Polisson R, Blotner S *et al.* (1993). The effects of drug therapy on radiographic progression of rheumatoid arthritis—results of a 36 week randomized trial comparing methotrexate and auranofin. *Arthritis Rheum* **36**:613–19.

Weinblatt ME, Coblyn JS, Fox DA *et al.* (1985). Efficacy of low-dose methotrexate in rheumatoid arthritis. *N Engl J Med* **312**(13):818–22.

Weinblatt ME, Kaplan H, Germain BF *et al.* (1990). Low-dose methotrexate compared with auranofinin adult rheumatoid arthritis. A thirty-six-week, double-blind trial. *Arthritis Rheum* **33**:330–8.

Weinblatt ME, Keystone EC, Furst DE *et al.* (2003). Adalimumab, a fully human anti-tumour necrosis factor monoclonal antibody for the treatment of rheumatoid arthritis in patients taking concomitant methotrexate. *Arthritis Rheum* **48**:35–45

Weinblatt ME, Kremer JM, Bankhurst AD *et al.* (1999a). A trial of etanercept, a recombinant tumor necrosis factor receptor: Fc fusion protein, in patients with rheumatoid arthritis receiving methotrexate. *N Engl J Med* **340**(4):253–9.

Weinblatt ME, Reda D, Henderson W *et al.* (1999b). Sulfasalazine treatment for rheumatoid arthritis: A meta-analysis of 15 randomized trials. *J Rheumatol* **26**:2123–30.

Weitoft T, Uddenfeldt P (2000). Importance of synovial fluid aspiration when injecting intra-articular corticosteroids. *Ann Rheum Dis* 59: 235.

Wells G, Haguenauer D, Shea B, Suarez-Almazor ME, Welch VA, Tugwell P (2000). Cyclosporine for rheumatoid arthritis. Cochrane Database Syst Rev: CD001083, Oxford.

Wenger ME, Alexander S, Bland JH, Blechman WJ (1983). Auranofin versus placebo in the treatment of rheumatoid arthritis. *Am J Med* **75**:123–7.

Willkens RF, Urowitz MB, Stablein DM, McKendry RLF, Berger RG, Box JH (1992). Comparison of azathioprine, methotrexate, and the combination of both in the treatment of rheumatoid arthritis. A controlled clinical trial. *Arthritis Rheum* **35**:849–56.

Willkens RF, Sharp JT, Stablein D, Marks C, Wortmann (1995). Comparison of azathioprine, methotrexate, and the combination of the two in the treatment of rheumatoid arthritis. *Arthritis Rheum* **38**(12):1799–806.

Williams JH, Reading JC, Ward JR, O'Brien WM (1980). Comparison of high and low dose cyclophosphamide therapy in rheumatoid arthritis. *Arthritis Rheum* **23**:521–7.

Williams HJ, Ward JR, Reading JC *et al.* (1983) Low-dose D-penicillamine therapy in rheumatoid arthritis. *Arthritis Rheum*, **26**:581–92.

Williams HJ, Willkens RF, Samuelson CO Jr *et al.* (1985). Comparison of low-dose oral pulse methotrexate and placebo in the treatment of rheumatoid arthritis. A controlled clinical trial. *Arthritis Rheum* **28**(7):721–30.

Williams HJ, Ward JR, Dahl SL *et al.* (1988). A controlled trial comparing sulfalazine, gold sodium thiomalate, and placebo in rheumatoid arthritis. *Arthritis Rheum* **31**(6):702–13.

Wolfe F, Mitchell DM, Sibley JT *et al.* (1994). The mortality of rheumatoid arthritis. *Arthritis Rheum* **37**:481–94.

Woodland J, Chaput de Saintonge DM, Evans SJW, Sharman VL, Currey HLF (1981). Azathioprine in rheumatoid arthritis: double-blind study of full versus half doses versus placebo. *Ann Rheum Dis* **40**:355–9.

Zerdler HK, Kvien TK, Hannonen P *et al.* (1998). Progression of joint damage in early active severe rheumatoid arthritis during 18 months of treatment: comparison of low-dose cyclosporin and parenteral gold. *Br J Rheumatol* **37**:874–82.

INDEX